Ellen M Bard

Your Work Wellness Toolkit

Mindset Tips, Journaling and Rituals to Help You Thrive

Ellen M Bard is a work psychologist, writer and speaker. She is on a mission to bring practical, useful and fun development suggestions and personal and professional improvement ideas to those who are long on interest and short on time.

Ellen is an Associate Fellow of the British Psychology Society, Chartered Occupational Psychologist and registered with the Health Professions Council (HPC) in the UK. She has published papers and spoken on topics including values in the workplace, leadership, being your best self at work, engagement, the candidate experience in recruitment, psychometric tools, generation Y and employer branding. She has been featured in the *Huffington Post*, *The Guardian*, BBC Radio 4 and the *Financial Times*, as a thought leader in productivity and the challenges of work–life balance.

In her 20-year career, she has worked in more than 25 countries, with people from over 40 countries, and after 12 years working in People Consultancies in Dublin, Ireland and London, UK, she moved to Bangkok, Thailand, where she has lived for the past eight years. Her work includes supporting organizations in areas such as development, training, assessment, recruitment and coaching, which has given her the experience and the passion to bring you stuff that really works.

Contents

Introduction

Final Thoughts
Acknowledgements
Further Reading

Introduction

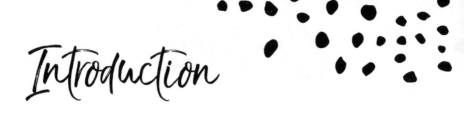

Do the Best for Future You

I lay in a hospital bed, drained, recovering from my first ever surgery. I had been admitted as an emergency the day before for acute abdominal pain, and the surgeon who operated on me had found a 4cm by 6cm cyst that had spread infection (and agony) throughout my abdomen.

She diagnosed me with endometriosis – my third chronic condition, to add to Crohn's disease and chronic pain from a car accident I had been involved in 20 years before. Oh, and there was a global pandemic raging around me, meaning I'd already had to entirely change the way I worked with clients in the past six months.

To say I was exhausted and feeling low would be an understatement.

I was halfway through writing this book, with the deadline approaching.

I needed to get well, and quickly.

The irony of needing to apply self-care and work wellness techniques so strongly to myself at this time was not lost on either me or my friends and family, who were quick to remind me of the need to practise what I preached.

Thankfully, I had 20 years of experience as a work psychologist to draw on, working with over a thousand individuals from 40 different nationalities on their development and helping them to be the best self they could be at work.

I rested, read, used gratitude techniques to think about all the wonderful things that were present in my life still (especially the invention of antibiotics, without which I would have died), reminded myself of my values and tried to focus on the things I could control rather than the things I couldn't. I journaled daily to process the challenging feelings that being diagnosed with a third chronic health condition brought up in me, and, after a couple of weeks, I was ready to get back to writing the book.

I used many more of the work wellness techniques you will find in these pages to support me as I did so, and writing the book grounded me in the idea of what it means to be truly well in the workplace, with all aspects of our lives flourishing.

It reminded me that investing time in being kind to ourselves when we're at work will pay off for "future us". The two weeks I took to rest and heal were necessary to ensure I was then in a good enough condition to get back to work as my whole-hearted self.

My "Hit-by-a-Bus" Moment

This is not to say it's easy to allow ourselves the time to take care of our wellness at work.

When I worked in a busy people consultancy in London, UK, I thought I was indispensable. I took on more and more work, working 50- or 60-hour weeks, trying to get everything done. My work was stressful and impacting negatively on my health, and though I didn't take time to look after my work wellness, I enjoyed my work, and I knew that the business needed me to achieve its goals.

I was wrong.

Suddenly, and with no warning, my father died of a heart attack at 55 years old. I was devastated, and I stopped work entirely for three weeks to support my mother and sister and help with funeral arrangements.

You will not be surprised to learn that my organization didn't fall apart without me. They were inconvenienced, but they coped. The tasks and actions that had been my responsibility were given to others, and when I came back three weeks later I was welcomed back with a shorter to-do list to settle me back in as I grieved.

This was my "hit-by-a-bus" moment, although it was an emotional, rather than a physical bus. Out of nowhere I stopped work (as if I'd been "hit by a bus") and went away for several weeks. My business had to carry on without me, and it did.

It reminded me that no individual is indispensable and, importantly, *that is a good thing*. Businesses will often accept us working harder and harder, but they don't want us to work so hard we burn out.

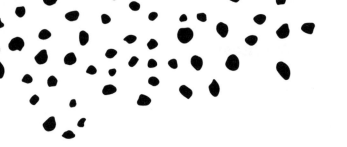

This applies to freelancers and small-business workers as much as employees in medium-size or large companies. If we don't keep ourselves healthy and well we are no good to anyone, as our work quality and quantity will be impacted. In fact, we run the risk of exhausting ourselves to the point where we can't work at all. We have to balance our desire to work hard because of the pressure to earn alongside taking the time we need to rest and recharge, so we can bring vitality and energy to our working lives.

Not only that, but while self-care is at the heart of work wellness, because it takes place in the work context, where we are naturally connected to others (whether they be colleagues, our boss, suppliers, clients or our wider professional network), when we invest time in many of the exercises in this book we are also likely to have a positive impact on the work wellness of those around us. When I was ill before the operation, it was harder for me to be kind and supportive to others, as all my energy went into managing my pain. Taking care of myself properly meant I had the vibrancy to engage with others in a way that aligned with my values, and to be a better version of myself.

What is Work Wellness?

Work wellness can seem like a contradiction in terms to some – "We're not at work to be kind to ourselves; we're there to do a job". Yet being our best self in the workplace helps us to do that job to the best of our ability.

Self-care is taking responsibility for our mental, emotional and physical health. While self-care in the context of work is at the heart of work wellness, it goes further than that, given our connections to those we interact with for work. The social and relational aspect of work wellness, and the environment we work in, also contribute to how we can flourish at work.

Work wellness is about taking action and responsibility for the issues we are able to affect. Too many of us feel passive in the work context, and while there are certainly things we can't change, we can do a lot about the way we approach the world and the choices we make. Work wellness progresses from "fixing issues" at work to being proactive so we can really thrive in the workplace.

Having said that, there are some things outside our control, and recognizing these also relieves some of the pressure on us. Burnout has recently been designated by the World Health Organization as a serious occupational health issue, in which chronic workplace stress has not been managed, and the individual experiences a state of emotional, mental and physical exhaustion.

Many factors can lead to potential burnout. The blur between work and personal life that has occurred due to technology and the need to work at home are factors that have increased levels of chronic stress in the working population.

The WHO's definition of burnout tells us that it is not only your issue to manage. Your organization bears responsibility as well, and as you understand how work affects you more, if you feel that you are approaching burnout, talk to your manager about the stress you feel they are putting you under; don't just go it alone. You can certainly do things to help you respond to the pressure your organization puts you under and how you feel about it, but the organization needs to step up as well, or it might be time for you to find a more supportive environment.

Work fits into our lives differently depending on whether we work in a large organization, a small company or we are self-employed. Additionally, our location impacts our work. Some of us work from home or cafés and co-working spaces, while others work in a dedicated office space. Others still are "hybrid workers" and their physical space changes depending on the day.

Wherever we work, for most of us work is very important. It takes up about a third of our lives, and it's worth investing time in it to make it work for us. Of course, the meaning of work isn't necessarily the same for everyone. Some people work simply to earn money, and the type of work they do is less important to them; they don't need it to be deeply meaningful. Others seek their "true calling" and passion, investing energy to make work purposeful.

Use the space below to brainstorm ideas on the following questions:

What does work wellness mean to you?

In what ways (if any!) are you currently kind to yourself at work?

What are the areas in which, or times when, you find it more challenging to keep yourself nourished in the workplace?

How to Use This Book

All the ideas in this book relate to any place that you set up your "office" –
from a physical location you go to every day, to your home office, to a café,
though you might have to adjust each idea slightly to each environment.
There's a chapter on some of the unique challenges of the home office, but
that doesn't mean all the ideas don't apply to both organizational offices
and home offices.

A key step in achieving work wellness is to get to know ourselves better.
Many of the ideas in this book will help you reflect on yourself, and as you
understand more your needs and boundaries, you can use the ideas to
help you thrive.

See all the ideas as experiments to try. Some will help you feel
nurtured and some won't resonate. That's not a problem. Everyone
is different, so pick what works for you and leave the rest. Be gentle
with yourself as you experiment, as this will help your self-care be
more sustainable. If you try to do everything at once, you may find
yourself overwhelmed.

A Note on Some Overarching Techniques

This book presents a collection of 100 ideas to support your work
wellness. It considers both your **physical environment** and the way you
interact with it, and it will help you to think about your work **mindset**,
to strengthen your understanding of yourself so you can engage with
work in the way that best suits you. It will consider the **home office** and
the unique challenges that brings us. It will help you make the most
of your **time** and **focus**, while balancing hard work with **breaks**. It will
remind you that even if you work alone, there is a **network of people
you can connect with**, and it will support you in **doing hard things**
and **managing change**. This book will help you grow and flourish,

and consider how and where to invest energy in your **personal and professional development**, so you can live the work life that enables you to prosper.

Rituals

Rituals can be simple or complicated, fanciful or practical. They can be repeated or one-offs. Don't be put off by the word – more and more research is being performed to examine how rituals in the workplace can boost performance and engagement.

They must be predefined (so don't make them up on the fly), meaningful to you and have some irrationality to them. Rituals help us by providing order and structure, even in situations where there might be none, which is calming to our brains. If you can tie the ritual into your core values, this will make it all the more powerful.

There are a number of suggestions on how to create rituals to support your work wellness in the book, but don't feel restricted by them. If there are other areas where you feel a ritual might benefit you, go for it!

Journaling

A number of the exercises will ask you to journal or free-write on key questions and ideas. This can be done in the book, on a computer or you can use a dedicated notebook – whatever works best for you. This toolkit has space for you to write answers in the book itself, but if you're a person who likes to write a lot, feel free to use an additional physical journal or notebook to log your answers so you don't feel constrained by space.

To journal, find a quiet space where you can reflect on the questions asked, and let the words flow. Use the timings given in the book as guides, but don't stop yourself if you want to write for longer. You never know what you might unearth when you pause and spend some time thinking.

CHAPTER 1

Physical Environment

Physical Environment

How does sitting at your desk make you feel?

We're starting our journey firmly in the environment that surrounds you: things you can touch, see or move around. We want to set up your physical workspace, whatever and wherever that may be, in a way that nurtures you and supports your wellness.

The right set-up for your desk can ensure you don't have physical issues that drain your energy but instead puts you in the best condition to do your work, wherever you may be doing that work, whether that be a formal office, at home, in cafés or anywhere else for that matter.

Our desk and the physical environment are areas many of us think about when we start in a role. We carefully place loved items on our shiny new workspace; we try out the settings of our chair; we take care to put our cups on a coaster. However, over time, our desk evolves without us noticing. We leave a pile of papers that we're going to get to at some point; the cups get put on that paper rather than a coaster and leave coffee rings; and clutter means we can't see the mementoes we included under the rubbish.

This chapter will help you to consider your desk and the environment around you with fresh eyes, and suggest both some one-off activities and some small habits you could include in your routine, so your desk feels like a place that supports you every day.

What you will find in this chapter

This is one of the most practical sections of the book, and the exercises are designed to prepare you to organize your work environment so that it fills you with joy and motivation, rather than acting as another drain on your energy. First you will **#1 Set Your Desk Up Right**, to make sure the tools you use are comfortable and don't create physical problems down the line. Then we'll look at including on your desk small tokens to help you **#2 See Beauty**, remind you **#3 You Are Loved** and that you can **#4 Look Forward** to your future even if there's a moment in your work day that's tougher than others to get through.

We'll consider the environment outside your desk area and how it impacts you, by thinking about what you need and can control in **#5 Your Soundscape**, as well as managing the environment in **#6 Blowing Hot and Cold**. We will also think about adding in some subtle scents to your environment so you can **#7 Use Your Nose** to manage the scents others produce that you may want to mask, or even to help you boost productivity.

We're not going to forget some basics, like **#8 Hydration**, as without this we may snack more or our performance might decrease. Another basic is to keep your tools clean and make sure you **#9 Wipe Down Your Technology**.

Lastly, we're going to learn how to **#10 Return to Neutral** at the end of the day, to ensure when we come back to our desk the next morning, we're not greeted with clutter that can deplete our energy before we even start work.

By the end of the chapter, you will have considered the physical environment that surrounds you and thought about how it can help you flourish despite traditional office, or newer, at-home challenges.

#1 Set Your Desk Up Right

Ergonomics is a word many of us aren't quite sure what to do with, but all we're doing here is ensuring our desk is comfortable enough that long hours of sitting don't exacerbate, or – worse – add physical symptoms, such as back or neck pain or sore wrists.

#23 Get Up and Move in the Working from Home chapter will also help support your physical health at work, but given you are likely to be sitting at your desk for many hours a week, it's worth the investment of time to set it up properly.

If you are at a big enough company, you may have a HR department that can assess this for you and provide you with the right equipment. For the rest of us, we need to make some more "homemade" adjustments. Note, these adjustments can still be made if you work from home or even in a café.

Review this list and tick the items when you've adjusted them:

☐ Chair – the chair height should mean your feet rest on the floor (or, as in the author's case, a firm cushion!). If your chair has armrests, your arms should be able to rest on these with shoulders loose. Don't slump; sit up tall on your sit bones (the bony parts of your bottom). The chair should support the curves of your spine – again, a cushion or lumbar support can help.

☐ Desk – make sure you can get your legs easily under the desk (be creative about raising the desk with bricks or wood if you need to).

☐ Monitor – keep the screen at or just below eye level, an arms-length away from your body.

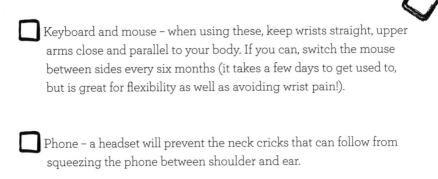

☐ Keyboard and mouse – when using these, keep wrists straight, upper arms close and parallel to your body. If you can, switch the mouse between sides every six months (it takes a few days to get used to, but is great for flexibility as well as avoiding wrist pain!).

☐ Phone – a headset will prevent the neck cricks that can follow from squeezing the phone between shoulder and ear.

If you use a laptop, you can still implement much of the above, or you can invest in a small separate keyboard and mouse, place your laptop on a stand (or pile of books!) and make the adjustments from there. This means that even if you're working from a café, or hot-desking at your kitchen table, there's no need to sacrifice your physical health.

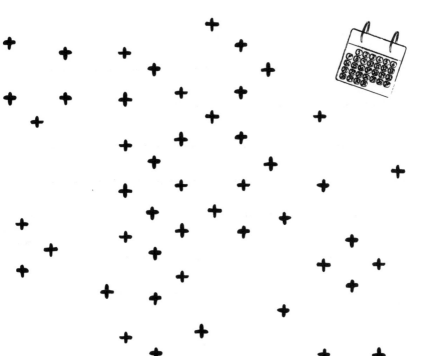

#2 See Beauty

A beautiful item is pleasurable to perceive and, by including beauty in our work lives, we can perk up our day by spending a minute or two every now and then contemplating such an item and reminding ourselves that there is a bigger, beautiful world out there. Perspective supports our work wellness.

Include on your desk something small and beautiful. This can be anything: a coaster, a shell, a photo or a pack of brightly coloured pens – whatever brings you visual joy.

Change the object with the seasons, or have several items in a drawer to swap in and out each month so you don't habituate and stop seeing the beauty right in front of you.

What object of visual beauty could you place on your desk?

_____

_____

Describe how you feel when you see the item.

_____

_____

What memories or associations does it hold?

_____

_____

#3 You Are Loved

While we're going to talk about nurturing your work relationships later in the book, we can also bring the love we feel outside the workplace into our work to keep us grounded.

Include on your desk something that reminds you that you are loved. This could be a photo of your child, parents, partner, a friend, pet or family member, a gift someone gave you or anything that brings you a warm sense that you are cared about when you really look at it.

Who are the five most important people in your life?

What item could you use to represent each of them?

1.
_____ ⟶ _____

2.
_____ ⟶ _____

3.
_____ ⟶ _____

4.
_____ ⟶ _____

5.
_____ ⟶ _____

Circle the one you will display first.

#4 Look Forward

Sometimes our work day is tough, and we need a little something to remind us that there are good things to come, even if working on this current report feels a bit like drudgery.

Having something that reminds you of future excitement can be a great way to re-energize and motivate you. This could be a sticky note with a word written on it that triggers the association, a coin from a country you will be visiting on holiday, the menu of a great restaurant you're getting take-out from at the weekend or a postcard from a friend who you're planning to have a video date with.

It's worth noting that if you're easily distracted or prone to daydreams, you might want to keep this item in your drawer (or your bag, if you're working in cafés) and get it out at times when you feel down, rather than having it on display all the time.

Name three things you are looking forward to in the medium term (1–6 months).

For each, write down something to represent a positive future that you could put on your desk.

I am looking forward to ...   What might represent this?

1. _____   _____

2. _____   _____

3. _____   _____

#5 Your Soundscape

Some people need quiet at work, while others like the hubbub of a noisy office. For others, the noise levels or types of music they might like depend on the task they are doing. There are even apps that provide music to help you focus on different tasks, or you can buy noise-cancelling headphones to remove some of the background noise in your office if it makes it hard to concentrate. Research suggests that music with lyrics is more likely to distract than to support, so the suggestion is to avoid that in the main as it takes up cognitive resources you'll need to spend on the work itself.

Write five types of task you do regularly and the kind of sounds/music – or lack thereof – that work best for you. For example, you might find that upbeat, no-lyrics guitar music is the perfect accompaniment to writing and responding to emails, while total silence is required for calculating your expenses. Don't be afraid to experiment!

Regular Task   Suitable Music (if any)

1.

2.

3.

4.

5.

#6 Blowing Hot and Cold

While air conditioning and central heating are a blessing, they can also play havoc with our internal temperature. A frigid environment can make it hard to work, while an environment that's too warm can be distracting and/or soporific.

Knowing what you need to cope with your environment and having this handy will help you to do your best work.

Fill in the table opposite with any items you need to have while working to manage the temperature – for example, socks, scarves, jumpers, moisturiser, contact lens eye drops or extra layers to add/remove as necessary.

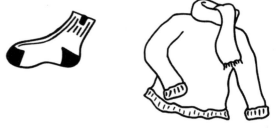

	Home office	Work office	Other space (1)	Other space (2)
Spring				
Summer				
Autumn				
Winter				

#7 Use Your Nose

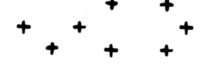

Whether our desk is in a café or a company office, even in our own home, most of us share the space we work in to some degree. That means that we likely deal with all kinds of sensory experiences that we don't necessarily choose. Just think of that all-too-common experience of someone heating up a microwave meal in the office, which then hangs around as an unpleasant smell all day.

Appropriate scents can improve mental clarity and evoke positive memories, and is an often forgotten but powerful tool in helping you be your best self at work.

Including scent into your work environment needs to be done carefully as, while you may love the smell of peppermint, it may make your co-worker sneeze. A few drops of perfume or essential oil on a cotton ball in a small plastic bottle or jar you can open and sniff works as well as anything else.

Below is a list of scents for that can boost productivity, according to research. Write down two ways you could access your chosen scent on your desk. (Remember, scent can be personal, so you might need to experiment to find what works for you.)

Peppermint: *Mint tea*   *Sucking mints*

Coffee: _ _ _ _ _ _ _ _ _   _ _ _ _ _ _ _ _ _ _

Rosemary: _ _ _ _ _ _ _ _ _   _ _ _ _ _ _ _ _ _

Lemon: _ _ _ _ _ _ _ _ _   _ _ _ _ _ _ _ _ _

Cinnamon: _ _ _ _ _ _ _ _   _ _ _ _ _ _ _ _ _

Pine: _ _ _ _ _ _ _ _   _ _ _ _ _ _ _ _ _

Note: Don't try all of these at once! Too many scents can be overpowering.

#8 Hydration

Often, when we think we're hungry, we're actually thirsty, and mild dehydration can give us a host of low-lying physical symptoms, including tiredness, headaches, light-headedness or difficulty concentrating.

Plan out what you typically drink in a well-hydrated day and make sure you set up reminders to hydrate, perhaps using an app or alarm on your phone or computer. It's also worth remembering that the amount of liquid you need is entirely personal and depends on the amount of exercise you do and what else you eat (there's water in food, too), so find the balance that works for you rather than following a "one-size-fits-all" rule.

Write down everything you typically drink in a work day (e.g. two coffees, three glasses of water, a ginger tea, a fruit juice, etc.).

Is this enough? Do you ever feel thirsty?

Are there times when you need to increase the amount you drink?

What are your strategies for making sure you don't forget to hydrate during the work day?

e.g. Water – fill an appropriately sized bottle at the start of the day, put it on my desk and make sure I drink it all.

#9 Wipe Down Your Technology

Our technology these days sees a lot of action. Sometimes we don't notice how grubby these items are (and potentially covered in germs) until the light strikes them just right, then, yuck! Make your technology easier on your eyes and less likely to be a source of germs by giving it a clean.

Cleaning can be a soothing activity, especially if you do it mindfully, giving it your full attention and making it a meditative activity.

Clean meditatively.

1. Gather your supplies (Make sure to check what you can/can't clean your technology with first! Suggestions might include a damp microfibre cloth and cotton buds.)
2. Turn your computer off.
3. Look at it for a moment. Consider all the amazing things this technology enables you to do – communicate with others, work, play, gather information etc.
4. Slowly and methodically clean your keyboard and screen, and any other part of the technology.
5. As you clean, pay attention to the movements and focus on your sensory experience.
6. Be present to each movement you make.
7. Once you are finished, take a deep breath and contemplate your technology.
8. Experience a moment of gratitude for everything it can do for you.

#10 Return to Neutral

At the end of each day, take a few minutes to return your desk to a "resting" state (this does not have to be minimalist, just clean and tidy). Throw away rubbish, put stationery back in its drawer or holder, neaten or put away papers, etc.

If you're lucky enough to have office cleaners, give them room to actually clean your desk. If not, run a wet tissue over the desk yourself. This will make coming in to work the next day a lot nicer.

Draw a picture of, or write about, what "neutral" would look like for your desk.

What feelings does this evoke?

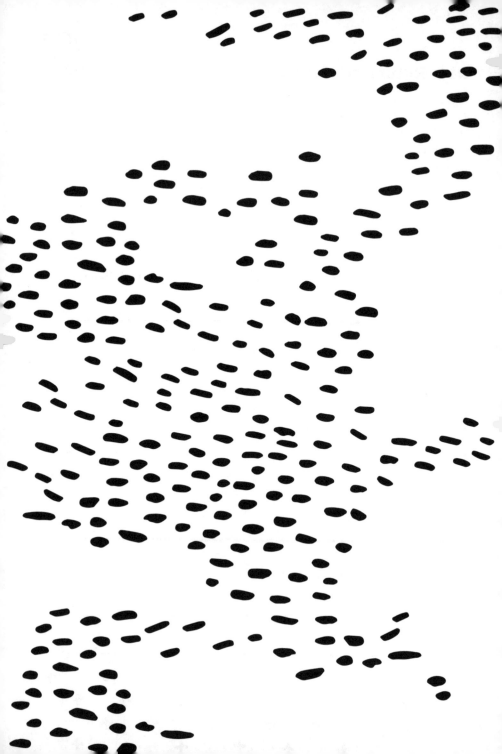

CHAPTER 2

Mindset

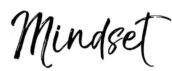

Mindset

Our mindset is the collection of assumptions, beliefs, ideas, values and other aspects that shape our way of thinking. In the context of work, our mindset can make or break a day.

All of us have underlying beliefs about work that are partly responsible for how we approach it, many of which we may not even be conscious of. For example, if we have the belief "we have to work hard to get ahead", we might distrust when a task comes more easily to us and believe that it's not a worthy achievement unless we suffered for it.

You can imagine your mindset as a piece of coloured glass through which you see the world. This filter gives you a certain perspective on things, while others might see through glass of a different colour. When we realize our mindset is one way of seeing the world, and that there are other possibilities, we can step back to make more deliberate choices about the coloured glass we see through – or we can try on others' glasses for size.

This deeper consideration of what we think about work gives us the opportunity to reassess the foundations on which we're basing our actions. We can be more conscious and deliberate in our choices in order to nurture ourselves at work from the inside out: how we approach our work makes a huge difference to how we feel about it, and this can create a virtuous or vicious circle depending on the mindset we choose.

What you will find in this chapter

We're going to review a set of tactical and strategic ideas around mindset to ensure that you're supported, rather than sabotaged, by your own brain.

We'll start with the practical, and ensure you include **#11 One Positive Interaction a Day** with others.

Then we'll go a bit deeper, and **#12 Name Your Work Why**, to think about the motivations behind why you work, and what you gain from the experience. We'll consider some of our coloured glass filters and help you **#13 Dig Up Your Beliefs About Work**, before we **#14 Shed a Negative Belief** that no longer serves you.

Next we'll get proactive and **#15 Choose Your Values**, before you **#16 Use Your Values** to guide decisions and help you find the path that's right for you in complex situations.

To support you, there are **#17 Three Ways to Remind You of Your New Focus**, so you can make sure you're putting your new mindset into practice every day.

We'll then **#18 Create a Start Ritual** and **#19 Create a Close Ritual** to give your day more purpose and help with better boundaries around work versus non-work time.

Lastly, we'll remind ourselves of the beautiful and wise **#20 Serenity Prayer** to help you focus your energy on what you can change, rather than wasting energy on issues that are outside of your control.

#11 One Positive Interaction a Day

Work can be a tough place where people are busy and focused on their own worries. We all have a bias toward the negative. This is because we evolved to be able to quickly notice dangers in the environment, while the positives of a situation fade more easily into the background.

What that hardwiring for survival means for us in our modern-day world is that we need to be active about noticing the good, and manage life so we have a far greater number of "positive" interactions than "negative" ones to ensure the negative doesn't take over – likely three to five positive interactions for every single negative interaction.

We can take steps ourselves to create an environment to increase our positive interactions, and help our mindset to be more enthusiastic about work by being proactive and trying to create at least one positive or kind interaction every day at work. In this way, our actions can also influence others – creating not just work wellness for us but for those around us.

Opportunities for creating positive interactions might involve:

- Smiling at others

- Greeting people positively when you see them in the morning

- Asking others how their weekend was

- Sending a quick message to someone in your network congratulating them on a new job or an achievement

- Praising someone for something small they've done for you or helped you with

- Affirming a positive behaviour

- Asking others what they're enjoying about their work right now

- Sharing a coffee or lunch with a colleague, giving them your full attention

Write down five positive interactions that you will attempt this week, one for each work day. Be specific with the person's name and what you will do. Remember, small acts are just as effective as big ones.

Monday _____

_____

Tuesday _____

_____

Wednesday _____

_____

Thursday _____

_____

Friday _____

_____

#12 Name Your Work Why

We all have different – usually multiple – reasons for working, each one personal to us.

We might work because we want to earn money and pay the bills, or enjoy the feeling of completion each day when we finish our shift. We may enjoy the social aspect of being around others and working in a team. We might like being creative or managing others or feel that our job is a "calling". Some of us work to earn enough money to live a great life outside work, while the work itself is of less importance. For others, the work itself is the critical thing and we will sacrifice other things, like comfort or financial security, to do the activities we love.

Identifying the reasons you work can help when it's hard to get up in the morning and switch on the laptop, or head to the office. Re-reading your reasons and reminding yourself can provide added motivation to get you going.

List the three main reasons you work:

1. _____

_____

2. _____

_____

3. _____

_____

#13 Dig Up Your Beliefs About Work

We all have a lot of beliefs about work – some of them helpful, others not
so much. These beliefs are our opinions and attitudes toward the work we
do, and they come from all sorts of sources in our past and present.

Without a bit of digging and examining, we may make decisions based
on an unexamined but, in truth, outdated belief. For example, just because
your grandfather told you when you were little that if work wasn't hard,
it wasn't real work, doesn't mean that's a belief you need to keep.

**Spend ten minutes thinking about all the things you believe about
work and write them here.**

*Examples: "Work is a chore"; "I only work to earn money"; "My work
should have a deeper meaning".*

How do these beliefs inform your attitude to work?

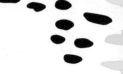

#14 Shed a Negative Belief

Some of the beliefs we have can be helpful, while others can foster unhelpful feelings or ideas about what we "should" be doing or what we "have to" do, and these can limit our personal growth and expansion.

In addition, the same belief can be positive for one person and negative for another. For example, "I only work to earn money" can be freeing for one person, as it means they can forget about work in their leisure hours, or it can be a chain for another, as it means they feel their job doesn't have any greater meaning, which is something they long for.

Identify one of your beliefs about your work life or your job that is causing you negative feelings and emotions and write it down.

_____

_____

Challenge your belief. Can you really say, without any doubt at all, that this belief is true? If you have any evidence to the contrary, write it down.

_____

_____

Where did this belief come from? (Don't worry if you don't know; sometimes the source is unclear.)

_____

_____

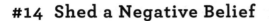

Write the statement "I choose not to believe [write the belief here] anymore." Read the statement aloud.

_____

_____

What belief would serve you better? Write this here. Read it aloud.

_____

_____

What evidence do you have for this new belief?

_____

_____

Put this new belief somewhere you will see it every day – for example, on a Post-it note on your desk, or set it as one of your passwords so that you type it daily.

Experiment with going about the world as if it were true.

#15 Choose Your Values

Once we've explored the current terrain of our work mindset through our beliefs and our "why", we can then look at creating values to guide our future actions and mindset.

A value is something that is important to us, something that can guide our actions and behaviour. Once you've chosen them, they can be like a compass. Whenever you need to make a decision, and you're uncertain, simply choose the path that is most aligned with your values.

Choose your values – the four most important principles in your life – and write them here.

Examples might be: kindness, freedom, delight, family, love, courage, health, financial security, open-mindedness, growth, adventure, loyalty, fairness, innovation, etc.

1.

2.

3.

4.

#16 Use Your Values

Now you have clarified your values, they can help you find meaning and alignment with your work, as you consider how your job reflects these values.

How does your work serve your values

_____

_____

_____

How could it serve or align with your values more deeply?

_____

_____

_____

What one action could you take for each value this week that would help you behave more in line with your values?

VALUE   ACTION

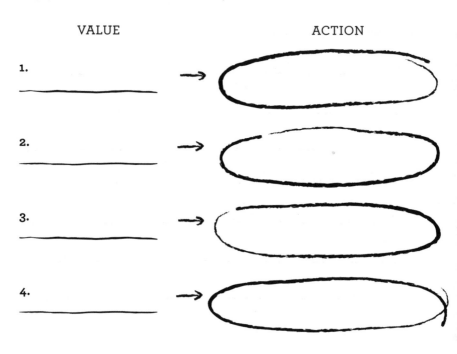

1. _____ →

2. _____ →

3. _____ →

4. _____ →

#17 Three Ways to Remind Yourself of Your New Focus

When you have a new habit or you want to remind yourself of something new or important, such as a value or a positive belief, there are several ways you can use your technology to your advantage to keep what you want to remember front of mind.

1. Use it as a password. (You just need to make sure you turn off the autocomplete option so you actually have to type the word or phrase every day!)

2. Make it your screen saver. (You could even have your screen saver cycle through multiple values.)

3. Use it as your screen background.

With any of these, change it up once every couple of weeks so you don't "habituate" and stop seeing whatever word or phrase you've chosen.

What will your reminder to yourself be?

#18 Create a Start Ritual

Being intentional in your approach to work can make a huge difference to your mindset, and creating a conscious, focused ritual to start and close the day can be a big contributor to work positivity.

It doesn't have to take a long time or include a lot of steps, but by creating something purposeful, with a few deliberate, repeated actions, you can condition your brain to approach work in the way you want, rather than just reacting to whatever happens and getting distracted by others' issues.

For example, a start ritual could involve:

- Taking a deep breath as you step over the threshold (whatever you consider that to be) of your workplace

- Greeting people with a smile as you walk to your desk

- Turning the computer on

- Going to the kitchen to get a coffee

- Settling at your desk and taking three deep breaths

- Reminding yourself of your "why" (**#12 Name Your Work Why**)

- Picking one of your values and writing it on a Post-it alongside a behaviour that will allow you to live that value today

- Starting work

Of course, if you prefer, you could just do the smile, coffee and deep breath! It's all about whatever works for you and what tells you it's time to start work, with the mindset you've chosen.

Write down 3–10 ideas for your own start ritual and then number each one to signify the order in which you will do them.

Try the start ritual for a week, then come back and answer the following questions:

How did it feel starting your day with this ritual?

What was missing?

What needs to change?

Revise the ritual based on your experience, if necessary.

#19 Create a Close Ritual

A close ritual is the reverse of the start ritual, and is a set of steps that tells your brain that you are done with work and can move to leisure (or whatever you are doing once work is done).

An example might be:

1. Check your email to make sure everything is dealt with and you don't have loose ends

2. Clear your desk and **#10 Return to Neutral**

3. Check in with your values and think about how you lived each of them today

4. Write down something you learned from your day

5. Take three deep breaths

6. Turn your computer off

7. Leave – with a smile for your co-workers!

Write down how you will purposefully "close" your day.

Pair it with your start ritual for the next two weeks.

After that, tweak both the start and close rituals to suit your needs.

#20 Serenity Prayer

"Grant me the serenity to accept the things I cannot change, courage to change the things I can, and wisdom to know the difference."

Serenity Prayer, Reinhold Niebuhr

Such wise advice contained in just one sentence.

We care about a lot of things, but we can't always change the things we worry about.

These words remind us that we are better off putting our energy into the things that our actions can influence, rather than investing energy into the things that we worry about but cannot change.

For example, we may worry about whether our boss will give us the promotion we want. But our boss's choices are her decision and outside our control. However, *our* choices of action *are* within our control. We can step up and take on harder projects, we can create positive change in our organization, we can do a great job on the projects we are given and we can look after our teams.

By shifting our mindset, we have more power to take proactive responsibility for the shaping of our lives, rather than be a powerless victim of circumstance.

Fill in the circles below.

In the inner circle, write issues you can do something about (for example, your own behaviour, actions, how you manage the expression of your feelings, how you treat others, how you stick to your promises, etc.).

In the outer circle, write issues over which you have no control (the actions of others, the feelings of others, workplace politics, etc.).

What in the inner circle can you take a small action on today?

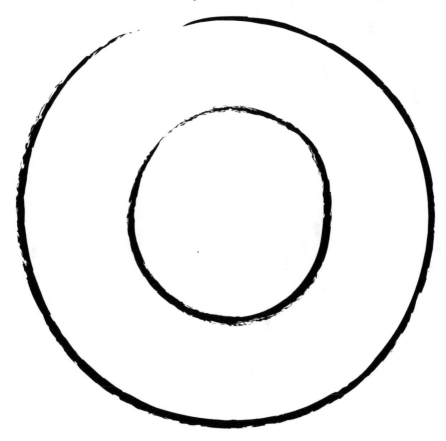

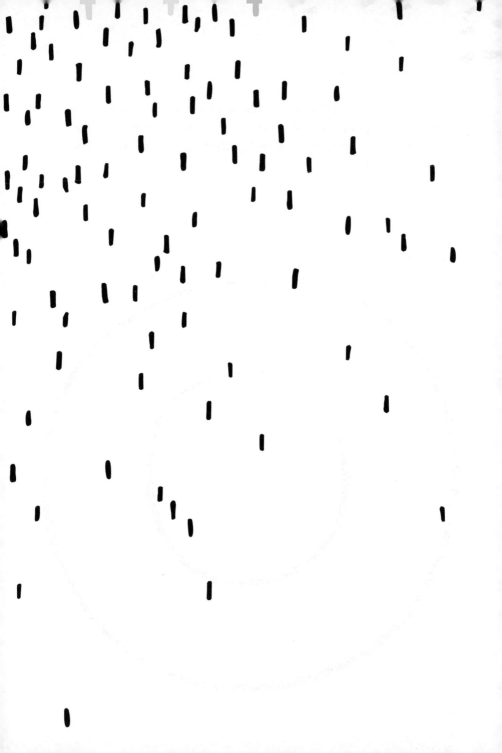

CHAPTER 3

Working from Home

Working from Home

While all the exercises and activities in this toolkit apply to working from anywhere, some special challenges can arise when working in a space that isn't a designated office environment. Having said that, while the emphasis is on the home workers, some of these exercises may still be useful if you're based in an office, so have a read through and take anything that works for you.

These days, hybrid working is in demand and on the rise. Employees want to be flexible enough to work where and when they want, whether that is remotely, at home or in person within an office set-up. This blended model of working creates challenges in both the physical and the digital worlds, but it can also create opportunity.

Many of us have had to devise "home offices" out of nothing, fitting them into a space that was already full of our non-work lives. We may find ourselves eating, working and socializing at the same table, and the boundaries between when we're working and when we're relaxing have become permeable.

We've become more vulnerable because it's harder to hide who we are at home from those we work with when it's on display in a video chat, but this also enables us to bring our authentic self to work – even though, it must be said, that self is often exhausted.

Equally, we're able to spend more time with family and friends when we have a commute that takes a minute rather than an hour.

What you will find in this chapter

In this section, we'll first try to understand how to **#21 Manage Digital Fatigue**, before it's time to **#22 Plan Your Meals** so you nourish yourself from the inside out. Ensuring we **#23 Get Up and Move** will also help our bodies support us through a working day that doesn't have the benefits of travelling between desks or rooms to visit and meet with others.

We'll put in clear boundaries between work and leisure through **#24 Thresholding** and make sure you **#25 Keep it Regular** by creating rhythms and routines that mimic those of an office, while allowing you the flexibility of working from home. You'll be better able to do this if you **#26 Know Your Distractions**.

Keeping our social connections alive while at home is critical to our wellbeing, so we will also look for ways to **#27 Replace Your Water Cooler Talk**.

Finally, we'll consider the huge role that video conferencing now plays in our lives, and make sure your **#28 Lights, Camera, Action: Input** and **#29 Lights, Camera, Action: Output** are conscious and help you to be a positive presence in others' work lives. We will end by thinking about **#30 What Messages Are You Sending?** to ensure you are showing off your best self to others.

#21 Manage Digital Fatigue

If working from home, you are likely to experience digital fatigue – mental exhaustion from the overuse of digital tools and technologies. We use multiple online tools for work and social needs, often at the same time. Many of the suggestions in this Working from Home chapter will help with this exhaustion, but decreasing your screen time and performing any activities you can offline will help your energy levels stay high.

Investing in pretty coloured pens and a pad of paper can pay dividends here. They can be used for making offline lists, note-taking, planning or even making brainstorming a more fun activity. If you can do some of these offline activities in the sun – in a garden, on a balcony, sitting by an open window or even out walking if you just need to think – it can help you feel replenished and revived.

What activities that you currently do online could you do offline?

_____

_____

_____

How could you make these offline activities more enjoyable and energizing?

_____

_____

_____

#22 Plan Your Meals

When we work at home we have access to a whole kitchen and, because we often use food as an antidote to boredom (or we fill up on food when we're actually thirsty – see **#8 Hydration**), it pays dividends to be prepared. So stock up on healthy snacks, think beforehand about approximately when and what you will eat each day, and stay hydrated.

Fill in the table below at the weekend or a couple of days in advance to make sure you have the ingredients in the house. By planning your meals like this, you're less likely to either be drawn down a time sink of wondering what you should eat or grabbing whatever seems easy or appealing at the time – which is usually not very healthy, as we tend to be more attracted to energy-dense foods like pizza or chocolate when we are hungry.

Write down some ideas for this week:

	Breakfast	Lunch	Dinner	Healthy snacks
Monday				
Tuesday				
Wednesday				
Thursday				
Friday				

#23 Get Up and Move

In the office, we tend to get up fairly often to do small errands – to ask a co-worker something, get a coffee, collect documents from the printer, etc.

While we're still likely to hit the kitchen while working from home, because the space is probably smaller, with fewer people around there aren't as many reasons to get up, so you may find yourself sitting more than ever, especially if you are no longer commuting. We have to remember that movement energizes our brain and allows for creativity to flow, so if you're feeling an energy slump, struggling to get motivated or stuck on your work tasks, get moving! It's like turning the key in the ignition to get you going again.

Set a timer on your computer (probably a silent, visual one if you have a lot of meetings – I appreciate it's not always possible to get up and walk off if you're in the middle of a video call) and get up once an hour for at least two minutes. Make sure you time the two minutes, too!

Movement doesn't have to be "exercise". Simply move your body in whatever way feels intuitive or good or put on a short song and dance to it. Once a day, at the start, end or during your lunch break, try to move for a longer time – do some cleaning, feed the birds, water the plants or take a quick walk.

Come up with five ways you can move your body for two minutes and list them here. Remember, it doesn't matter what, as long as they get you up from your desk.

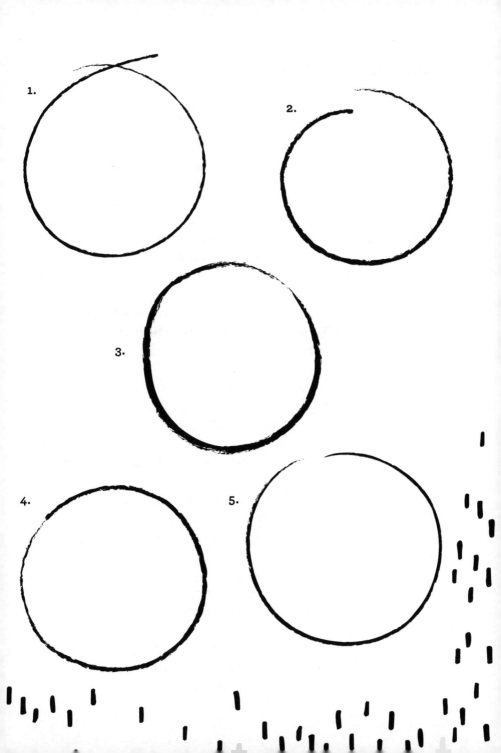

#24 Thresholding

A huge challenge of working from home is the lack of boundaries or "thresholds" between our work and leisure time. We can find ourselves working late without noticing, or elongating our work day by playing a quick game (or seven) of Candy Crush during work time in the knowledge that we can always make up the time at the end of the day.

Having clear boundaries to tell ourselves when it's work time and when work time is over can make a big difference to our overall work wellness, both in terms of our productivity within the work day and our ability to better enjoy and be refreshed by our leisure time.

You can use a start or close ritual (see **#18 Create a Start Ritual** and **#19 Create a Close Ritual**) or even **#10 Return to Neutral** to help with this, but thresholding can be much simpler.

Pick one small action to do and at the end of that action say (ideally aloud), "Now I am at work." At the end of the day, do the action in reverse, and say (again, aloud), "Now I have finished work."

The action at its simplest can be literally stepping between the thresholds of home and work, such as into a home office. Alternatively, it could include a five-minute walk out of the house that acts like a commute, so you are able to step back into the house (or coffee shop, etc.) in the morning "at work", or into the house after work in the evening to signal the beginning of "leisure time".

You could even try putting on slightly smarter clothes in the morning and changing these for something more casual in the evening.

Alternatively, your action might be a 3–5 minute breathing meditation, where you focus on the words "Now I am at work" and "Now I have finished work" depending on which is relevant.

As always, the choice is yours – experiment to find something that suits you.

Write down three possibilities to experiment with thresholding.

At the start of the day I will:

1.

2.

3.

At the end of the day I will:

1.

2.

3.

#25 Keep it Regular

When we work in a physical office, we're somewhat bound by its rhythms. Typically, we're "expected" to show up at a certain time, leave after a certain number of hours and take breaks at set points during the day.

When we work at home, unless our days are endless video meetings, our schedule can be a lot more flexible – which has its pros and cons. We forget sometimes that routine can be helpful. For one, it can take the pressure off having to make decisions at every moment about what's next. For another, when we've already consciously made decisions about our activities, they won't be affected by our emotions or moods in the moment.

Routine doesn't mean doing the same thing every day, or having your life planned out to the minute. It could mean some set activities each day – e.g. your start time, finish time and a period during which you have lunch – or it could mean always starting your week with a team meeting, and ending it with a review of the week.

Journal for 20 minutes on the following questions:

What aspects of your work have to be consistent for you each week?

What aspects do you enjoy being consistent each week?

Do you have an approximate start and finish time for your work?

Do you have an approximate time you take food or rest breaks during the day?

Are there things you should do more often in a week?

Are there things you should do less often in a week?

Your answers to these questions can help you to think about creating a home-office rhythm and balancing that endless (and sometimes exhausting) flexibility, without losing the benefits.

#26 Know Your Distractions

We all have things that pull us away from work. To start with, we check our phones on average 160 times a day – and many of these instances will be out of mindless habit or the pull of a needless notification.

As ever, the more we know ourselves, the more we can manage things proactively. Likely distractions to watch out for include habitually and unnecessarily checking emails, procrastinating from a task by making a snack, watching TV, checking your social media, etc.
Tips for overcoming these distractions include:

- Turning off notifications during certain periods of the day
- Using an app blocker on your phone so you can only check social media out of office hours
- Working in a different room from your phone
- Logging out of apps when you're not using them at work

Today, keep a journal of every time you find yourself pulled out of your intended work to do something else that you didn't plan.

What distractions recur? Consider how you can reduce or remove that distraction using the tips above

#27 Replace Your Water Cooler Talk

The office environment provides a casual social network that we almost don't notice – until it's gone. When we're at home, especially if we live on our own, we may miss creating the bonds with our workmates that come from chats about last night's TV, or how their cat is – connection for connection's sake. Humans, as social animals, need those interactions, and when we work at home our focus can get in the way. Finding a way to replace this "water cooler talk" can be invaluable.

At the start of every one-to-one work call, plan out three questions to ask the other person (not the same ones every time!). This demonstrates an interest in them and hopefully they will reciprocate. This might have the added benefit of others seeing you as a human with a life outside work and, equally, you can empathize with some of the non-work challenges others are going through. This can make it easier if you need to **#99 Handle Non-Work Issues** at some point.

Write out ten possible questions you can ask people at the start of a call.

Example: How are you doing?
What are you working on at the moment?

1.

_____

2.

_____

3.

_____

4.

_____

5.

_____

6.

_____

7.

_____

8.

_____

9.

_____

10.

_____

#28 Lights, Camera, Action: Input

Video calling is now a part of most of our lives and, while on the one hand it's pretty amazing, it has its downsides and brings new types of work fatigue.

By making some small tweaks, however, you can make this activity work better for both you and your colleagues.

Having your camera feed on at all times while on calls is like someone following you around with a mirror so they can see every movement as you make it. This is hugely distracting and stressful – and also unnecessary!

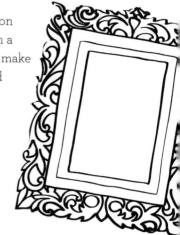

Instead, buy a hand mirror or use your phone to check before each call that there's no spinach in your teeth. Then, once the call has started and you've checked your camera is focused on your head, rather than your chest, hide "self-view".

Journal for 3 minutes on how it felt to do a call without the self-view on. What did you notice?

#29 Lights, Camera, Action: Output

If you've ever been on a video call where the other person was hard to hear or difficult to see, you'll know how annoying it is – and how much it can affect your perception of what they said. Do yourself (and your personal brand) and others a favour by investing in some low-cost, reasonable-quality technology – a microphone, headphones and a small selfie light. You'll feel brighter and better and it will help you shine.

Identify where you might benefit from an upgrade to your technology.

Research what's the best quality you can have in your budget – it's likely to be tax deductible! – or check with your employer if they will pay for it.

Play with the settings of your new technology. Write notes on what works best here:

_____

_____

_____

How do you feel looking at your "new self" in the camera?

_____

_____

_____

#30 What Messages Are You Sending?

Having taken part in a lot of video calls, I'm often surprised at the subconscious communication others send out through their choice of background. While some backgrounds can humanize you (I'm remembering the CEO who took part in a coaching call with me in his daughter's room because all the rooms in his house were busy, during which I spent the call trying not to look at the stuffed glittery unicorn on the shelf behind him), others can make you seem careless, childish, untidy, etc.

Journal for 20 minutes on the following questions:

What is the current background you have for video calls?

agine the background from a stranger's perspective. What might y about you?

What can you change physically? (At the most basic, a clean white sheet hung neatly over clutter might be worthwhile.)

Do you know how to apply a digital background? (Search engines can help.)

Experiment with changing the background. How do you feel about changing it?

What is the balance for you between "showing personality" and "showing professionalism"?

CHAPTER 4

Doing the Hard Stuff

Doing the Hard Stuff.

All of us have bad days at work or situations when things go "wrong". Dealing with these gracefully and managing their impact on you and the people around you is a core, if perhaps advanced, skill in terms of your work wellness.

In this chapter we consider some of the common work issues you might face that can create the most stress and anxiety. The tools in the Handling Change chapter may also support you with these. Either way, we will likely need to be gentle with ourselves when dealing with these kinds of issues. We should also remember that we are human along with our colleagues, and that we all face these challenges at one time or another. We're not alone.

What you will find in this chapter

In this section we will consider the role of mistakes at work, both in terms of **#31 How to Rectify a Mistake: Acknowledge it** and **#32 How to Rectify a Mistake: Make it Right**. We'll build on this by considering **#33 How to Learn from a Mistake**.

We'll think about how to find more delight and engagement **#34 When You Don't Enjoy Your Work**, and we'll also consider **#35 Imposter Syndrome: Create a Confidence Ritual** – another example where our emotions and brain can give us a skewed perspective, and where checking the evidence will help balance out that perspective.

Of course, sometimes we're actually not achieving what we want to in our job and that's when you'll want to think about **#36 When You're Not Performing Well: Role Model** to give you ideas on how you might improve. The next step is then **#37 When You're Not Performing Well: Honest Talk With Your Manager**.

Next we're going to get practical and consider the more boring, but very important, aspect of work wellness to **#38 Understand Your Benefits**. This is critical to your future self, and looking after your health and wellbeing in the long term.

Finally in this chapter we'll consider the very serious issue of **#39 Burnout** and what you might do to avoid this, as well as **#40 Knowing When and How to Leave** – a difficult decision but, every now and then, the right one to help you flourish.

#31 How to Rectify a Mistake: Acknowledge it

When we make a mistake at work, it's critical we take responsibility for our error. We also need to remember that everyone makes mistakes and, in the long run, your honesty will show others you can be trusted even when things are difficult. Getting more comfortable admitting your mistakes will help you manage these uncomfortable situations with grace.

Tips when acknowledging a mistake:

- Be clear that you understand you made a mistake. Say the words "I'm sorry". Don't add a "but"!

- Be specific. Say what it is you are apologizing for.

- Acknowledge the impact your actions caused and any possible consequences you can see.

- Repair. State what you are going to do to fix things. Ask for help if you need it.

Overall – keep it short and don't offer excuses.

Here is an example template:

"I'm sorry I [insert mistake here]. This means [insert consequence] and it might mean [insert consequence]. I intend to [insert what you will do to repair the mistake], but would it be possible for you to help me?"

I'm so sorry that I was late with the Kaynes Report by half a day. I've finished it now, but would it be possible for you to read my apology email to the client to ensure we keep the relationship?

Journal on a situation when you either did or didn't admit a mistake.

Situation:

_____

_____

What happened?

_____

_____

What did you do?

_____

_____

What was the impact?

_____

_____

Why did/didn't you acknowledge the mistake?

_____

_____

Write out an acknowledgement you could have used:

_____

_____

#32 How to Rectify a Mistake: Make it Right

Making a mistake at work can be mortifying and hugely anxiety-provoking. We think it will be a stain on the rest of our career and our first instinct might be to hide and hope it goes away. Well, real talk: it probably won't.

Taking ownership for a mistake, while difficult, is more likely to create trust with others in time. Idea **#31 How to Rectify a Mistake: Acknowledge it** is connected to and part of this – owning up to and apologizing for a mistake is the first part of making it right.

The second part is taking action to fix the situation as best you can, and this is obviously dependent on what the mistake was.

Did you miss a deadline? Talk to your boss about what you can do to get the work done as quickly as possible, and what message needs to go to the person whose deadline you missed and how.

Were you rude to a colleague? A simple apology might be enough.

Did you forget to do something? Be honest, apologize and tell them when you will do the task.

Write down two mistakes made recently by other people you know, and what they did to make it right:

Mistake:

How they made it right:

What else could they have done?

Mistake:

How they made it right:

What else could they have done?

#33 How to Learn From a Mistake

Seeing mistakes as learning opportunities helps to put them into perspective and makes them feel useful rather than shameful.

In order to learn from your mistakes:

1.   Engage with your mistakes consciously, considering how to fix them

2.   Review them after the dust has settled and draw out things you could do differently next time

3.   Apply these lessons in the future

Think of any (big or small) mistakes you have made in the past three months and then name an improvement you could make for each to deal with a mistake in future.

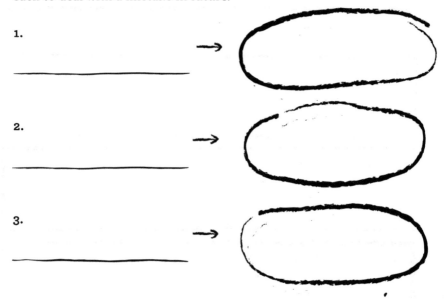

1.

→

2.

→

3.

→

When you next make a mistake, come back to this page and see if you can tweak your response on the basis of what you have learned in the past. You might then like to journal a second time on what you did differently based on your learnings and what impact it had.

Mistake one – what could I do differently next time?

_____

_____

_____

Mistake two – what could I do differently next time?

_____

_____

_____

Mistake three – what could I do differently next time?

_____

_____

_____

#34 When You Don't Enjoy Your Work

A difficult situation occurs when we're doing a role we're not enjoying. It impacts our motivation, we engage less with the tasks as well as with those around us, we may do worse at the job and then our morale lowers further. It's a vicious circle that amounts to the opposite of work wellness!

While finding a new job can be an answer, it's not always practical and instead we need to find the joy in what's in front of us.

Find your job description, and journal on the following:

What do you like about your job?

. - - - - - - - - - - - -- - - - - - - - - - -- - - - -

. - - - - - - - - - -- - - - - - - - - - -- - - - -

What don't you like about your job?

_____

_____

How close is what you currently do to what you were hired for?

. - - - - - - - - - - -- - - - - - - - - - -- - - - -

Are there activities you are doing that aren't in your job description and you don't like which you can let go of?

_____

_____

What are you really good at?

_____

_____

How else could you contribute to the team using your strengths?

_____

_____

What else could you get out of your job that's not about your core work? (Friendships, social activities, training, etc.)

_____

_____

If there is a very demotivating task or aspect of your job could you talk to your manager about how to make it more motivating?

_____

_____

What two actions can you take after this reflection?

Action 1:

Action 2:

#35 Imposter Syndrome: Create a Confidence Ritual

The first action to take when you feel you're not performing well is to check how true your feeling is. Imposter syndrome strikes when we achieve something, get praise and all we can think is *if only they knew what I'm really like*!

There's a disconnect between what others say about us and how we feel about ourselves. We feel like we're a fraud, an imposter and accolades and positive feedback only create more anxiety and doubt.

When we feel we're not doing well, the first step is to check feedback from others. Compare **#82 Assess Your Own Development Needs** with **#83 Get to Know What You Need to Develop**, and see if what others say echoes how you feel. If there is a disconnect, consider the idea that you may be suffering from Imposter Syndrome.

#84 Keep a Success File to remind you of the positive contribution you make to work – include complements you've received, successful projects you're proud of and endorsements you've had from people you respect and admire.

Create a Confidence Ritual to ground you in what's real. This could include some deep breathing, reading some of your success file, getting in touch with your senses one by one, feeling gratitude for your strengths, naming a number of them aloud and listening to an upbeat, positive song. Whatever works!

Create your personal Confidence Ritual. Write the steps opposite. Use this ritual when you're feeling a disconnect between how you feel about yourself and how others tell you they see you.

My Confidence Ritual

_____

_____

_____

_____

_____

_____

_____

_____

_____

_____

_____

_____

_____

#36 When You're Not Performing Well: Role Model

Sometimes we're really not performing well in our job, which can feel demotivating and uncomfortable. When performance issues become a longer-term trend rather than individual instances, we need to get proactive. This activity looks at how we can start by handling it alone, and **#37 When You're Not Performing Well: Honest Talk with Your Manager** is about getting help.

Step one in either of these situations is to understand where you're not doing well. What feedback have you had from others? Is your performance suffering in a specific area? A type of behaviour? What kind? Communication? Planning? Relationships with others? Report writing? Use idea **#83 Get to Know What You Need to Develop** if you don't already have a good idea, and try to pin it down to specifics.

Once you've understood where you need to perform better, identify someone who is really good at your problem area (you don't need to let them know).

Then play at being a detective-psychologist: create a mind map or set of notes detailing what they actually do that means they are great at this. Include behaviour, actions, body language, choice of words, how they interact, how they come across to others – be as specific as possible.

Break these behaviours down into chunks that you can experiment with in your own work.

```
┌─────────────────────────────────────┐
│                                     │
│            My Road Map              │
│                                     │
│                                     │
│                                     │
│                                     │
│                                     │
│                                     │
│                                     │
│                                     │
│                                     │
│                                     │
└─────────────────────────────────────┘
```

What behaviour will I try this week?

- -

Keep a learning journal or log to keep track of which behaviour you try, and when, on whom, and the impact it has. Always ask yourself afterwards: "What will I do differently to improve things next time?"

```
┌─────────────────────────────────────┐
│                                     │
│           Learning Log              │
│                                     │
│                                     │
│                                     │
│                                     │
│                                     │
└─────────────────────────────────────┘
```

#37 When You're Not Performing Well: Honest Talk with Your Manager

Sometimes, we can see we're not doing well at work and nothing we do seems to have an effect. This might mean it's time to talk with your manager to get feedback and advice on what to do to improve (better to be proactive and talk to them before they talk to you).

Depending on what your relationship with them looks like, this can be harder or easier. Either way, the more you prepare for the talk, the better.

Example conversation:

Hi Manager, I wanted to talk to you because I'm struggling with report writing and I want to improve. I've taken the course on spelling and grammar, and I've read some example reports, but my work is still getting a lot of negative feedback from the report reviewers. I'm ready to invest more time in improving, but I'm a bit stuck on what else to do. Can you help?

Write ideas on your own script here and think about how you might position it.

- Opening introduction with context about the situation

- What you're struggling with

- What you've done so far

- Ideas you have on how you could do more

- Asking for help

- Agreeing next steps and a follow-up meeting

My Script

#38 Understand Your Benefits

When we accept a job, we usually look at the benefits offered, but many of us forget about them after this. As a result, we can miss opportunities, forget to put money into our retirement fund and, for many people, it feels stressful to engage with this area. This applies to self-employed people too, who can miss tax credits or other perks of being self-employed they might not have explored.

While this one might seem a bit mundane, it's the tough love sort of self-care – looking after yourself in the longer term. Remember, even if it seems boring now, Future You will be grateful!

What potential benefits are available to you, either in your work "package" or as a self-employed person?

Check back with your contract, talk to HR or your boss or consult colleagues or other self-employed people to make sure you don't miss anything. You might be surprised at what's on offer (financial, retirement, social, training, discounts, etc.).

List all the benefits here:

_____

_____

_____

_____

_____

_____

Which benefits are you going to prioritize taking up?

_____

_____

_____

_____

_____

#39 Burnout

Sometimes feeling rough at work is more serious than just not liking your job. It might be that your job isn't good for you and you've lost your motivation in a deeper way.

Burnout is recognized by the World Health Organization as an occupational condition, where workplace stressors have become chronic. You may have burnout/be burning out if you:

- Feel consistently exhausted

- Feel negative or cynical about your job

- Are becoming less effective at your role

Burnout is a challenge to deal with on your own because it is caused by the workplace culture around you, combined with your relationship to work. While many of the ideas in this book can help mitigate burnout or stop it becoming a full-blown syndrome for you, there also may be aspects of the work culture that are driving burnout, particularly pressure to work all the time, and you might not have control over those.

This means the workplace and stressors in the environment need to be addressed, rather than the focus being entirely on you changing your approach. If the environment doesn't change, you may need to think about leaving, in which case see **#40 Knowing When and How to Leave**.

Take time to pause. Get away from work, ideally somewhere with nature, and spend some time thinking and journaling.

> How do you feel about your job?

> Do you exhibit all three signs mentioned previously?

> Is it difficult to get out of bed? Are you struggling with daily life? Are you on the verge of tears all the time? Or do you feel that it's difficult for you to carry on?

In the circumstances above, your work wellness has taken a severe hit and it's time to get professional help, just as you would for a sore throat or a physical pain with no apparent cause. See your doctor and ask them to recommend a therapist.

In addition, talk to your manager about the demands your environment is putting on you. You can't do everything, and as we discussed in the introduction, if you were hit by a bus, they'd find someone to manage your workload. The business will almost certainly carry on with or without you.

If you're self-employed, it can feel more difficult with bills to pay and the responsibility falling solely on you to earn money. On the plus side, you're the one who's creating the work culture, so you have more power to change it.

#40 Knowing When and How to Leave

While there's a great deal we can do to make our work environment better, and to engage with our work more positively, there are sometimes situations, as in **#39 Burnout**, where it's time to move on and change job, or if you're self-employed, stop working with a specific client.

To decide if that time has come, we need to think about how we feel about our work and the impact it has on us.

Whether or not we are good at our job is only one aspect of whether or not the organization we work with is right for us. We also need to consider if we are able to live and express our values through our work with the organization and if we "fit" with the culture.

Once we decide to leave, even if we have negative feelings about our work, it's important for our long-term career wellness to leave on a positive note.

This involves giving appropriate feedback if asked. Rather than spewing everything awful that has happened over the past however many years, try to give balanced feedback, considering what the key messages might need to be. Hand over projects and tasks in a professional manner and, most importantly of all, maintain the relationships you have built. Leave on good terms, as you never know who you may come across in future workplaces.

How do you feel about your work?

On a scale of 1 to 10, where 1 is "not at all" and 10 is "I want to leave today", how would you rate your desire to leave the job you are in? Circle the number that applies to you on the scale below.

1   2   3   4   5   6   7   8   9   10

What other activities in this book, if any, could you do to decrease
your desire to leave?

1.

2.

3.

4.

5.

If your desire to leave is at 8 or above, make a plan to leave
gracefully. What would you need to do to exit on a positive note?

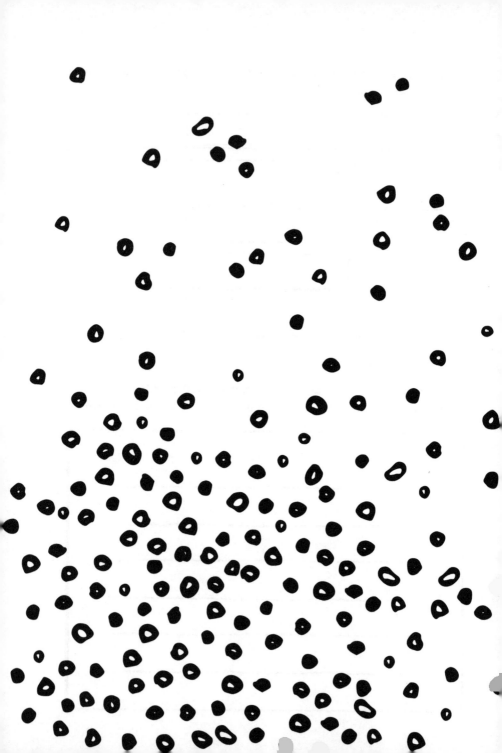

CHAPTER 5

Productivity and Focus

Productivity and Focus

Productivity isn't just about being busy all the time; it's about focusing on getting the important things done in a way that feels good. It's not about slogging away painfully, but about enjoying our work and producing a quantity and quality of activity that is expected by those who employ us (or that sometimes exceeds those expectations, but not by too much).

While there will always be some tasks that are less engaging than others, there are tweaks we can make to our environment to help us enjoy and engage more with the important work we do, allowing us to feel the sometimes elusive but absorbing state of "flow".

What you will find in this chapter

In this chapter, we start with **#41 Use Your Tech for You Not Against You**, by removing some of the digital noise that we are exposed to – for good. In **#42 Pull the Plug**, we turn off the remaining digital noise for short periods, and combine this with **#43 Use Pomodoros**, a simple method of including timed chunks of work for you to focus on.

We then ask **#44 Where Would You Like to Flow?**, and consider which of your tasks and activities might be the ideal place to focus on finding more productivity. Then it's time to **#45 Ready, Set, Flow** and create your own flow ritual, to put all these building blocks in place so you can enjoy the flow state more often.

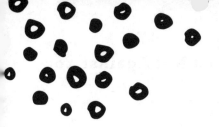

In **#46 Do You Really Need To?**, we will question whether all meetings were created equal, and then learn how to **#47 Subtract, Don't Add**, where you'll contemplate the removal of activities that aren't adding value to your day. We'll also ensure you have the tools to **#48 Limit the Scope** of the activities you do take on, so they don't become too much for you to handle.

Finally, we will split your time into **#49 Doing Time versus Deciding Time**, a tweak that can make quite a difference to procrastination. We'll then build on this by making sure you **#50 Set Goals You Can Actually Achieve**.

All these ideas will support your productivity and focus in a way that feels positive and helps you focus on the work that's really important.

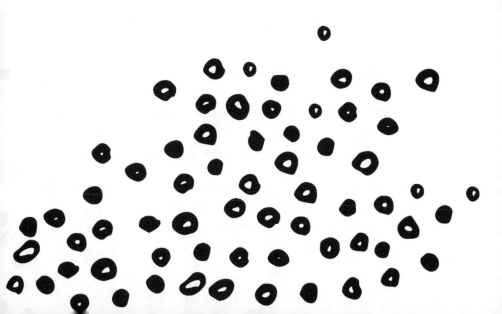

#41 Use Your Tech For You Not Against You

Many of us let our technology rule us. We allow the constant red dots and alerts to knock us off balance when we're doing a task, and we let information coming through our phone or computer take precedence over what we're doing – the tyranny of the supposedly "urgent" over the important.

Statistics for 2021 tell us that people have around 80 apps installed on the average smartphone, yet they use only nine of these per day and an average of 30 per month. This information give us a useful rule of thumb: you don't want more than about a quarter of your apps sending you annoying notifications, given you're not likely to be using the rest very often. Of course, that doesn't mean you can't choose to go in and check them when it's convenient to YOU.

1.   Count the total number of apps you have.

2.   Work out what 25 per cent of your total number of apps would be.

3.   Remove notifications from all but 25 per cent of your apps.
     *For example, if you have 80 apps on your phone, 25 per cent of
     these would equal 20 apps, so you would turn off notifications
     on 60 apps.*

After two days, come back and journal:

How do you feel with a smaller number of notifications turned on?

#42 Pull the Plug

We're rarely without our devices these days, yet the constant interruptions technology offers can greatly disturb our ability to concentrate.

When you really need to focus, unplug, mute or turn off your devices. If you're working on a computer, consider if you really need the internet turned on or whether you can work offline.

You'll likely feel the "pull" to check your devices: feel it, but don't give in to it. You can put the device in another room if you're struggling.

The world won't end if you don't check your email or phone notifications for 30 minutes, but your concentration will improve over time with this practice, helping you to achieve more.

Try a short period (20–30 minutes) in which you unplug.

How did it feel?

What apps or webpages did you feel most drawn to check?

What was most challenging for you about the experience?

Did you miss anything truly important during that 30 minutes?

#43 Use Pomodoros

Another tool to help us focus and concentrate, the Pomodoro Technique®
suggests we use a timer to break down our tasks into blocks – traditionally
25 minutes long – and then give ourselves a short break before we start
another timed block. (The technique was named after the tomato-shaped
kitchen timer that the inventor, Francesco Cirillo, used to break down the
time in blocks.) Keep track of the "pomodoros" by putting a checkmark on
a piece of paper, and after four pomodoros plus short breaks, take a longer,
30-minute break.

If you combine pomodoros with **#42 Pull the Plug**, you may find it easier
to start on difficult tasks, as you know you'll get a break from them in a
short time. Having a set time for the task helps concentration and, if you're
distracted during the pomodoro, you can remind yourself that you have
a break coming up to check TikTok or play with whatever is pulling your
attention away from the task.

Try two pomodoros of 25 minutes with a five-minute break in between.

How was it?

How did you feel focusing on one only thing for that period of time?

What was the impact on your concentration?

How did the break help/hinder your progress?

#44 Where Would You Like to Flow?

When we feel flow, we are energized by, absorbed in and fully enjoying the activity we are doing, and we lose track of time. Flow state has been linked to greater happiness and better emotional regulation.

Three conditions need to be met for us to achieve flow state in any task:

1. The activity must have structured, clear goals and the opportunity to progress. (*For example, writing a ten-page report on a certain topic by a certain time.*)

2. The task must be able to provide clear and immediate feedback for you to adjust your performance effectively. (*For example, you've written four pages of your report.*)

3. There needs to be a balance between how we perceive the challenges and how we perceive our abilities in the area, i.e. we need to feel confident that the task will stretch us but is still achievable. (*For example, the report is on a new topic, but you've written similar reports before.*)

Flow activities can be very varied, but are often found in sport, music, video games or the workplace – the latter being where we will focus.

Identify an area of work that is important to you in which you would like to achieve flow.

__ __ __ __ __ __ __ __ __ __

__ __ __ __ __ __ __ __ __ __

Remember, the area you choose needs to provide clear goals, immediate feedback and should stretch your skill level slightly but not too much as compared to the task.

#45 Ready, Set, Flow

Now you've chosen an area where you want to achieve flow, we're going to create a short ritual to set you up for flow. Repetition is a key part of telling your brain it's time for a certain type of activity, so once you've worked out your ritual, follow it each time you're ready to start a potential flow-finding activity.

For example, my flow ritual to start creative work is as follows, and I have it written on a Post-it on my laptop screen. Note: it's very practical!

1. *Tidy desk*

2. *Get a glass of water*

3. *Turn off email*

4. *Shut down all programs apart from those I am using to do the work*

5. *Put a certain type of music on, using headphones*

6. *Set a timer for 25 minutes*

7. *Silence and flip over my phone*

8. *Begin*

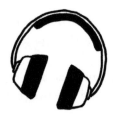

What short steps could you take as a flow ritual before you start
your flow activity?

How will these steps help you get into flow?

#46 Do You Really Need To?

We have a lot of meetings and calls for work, and we don't always question whether we personally need to be at them or even if the meeting itself is useful.

Can you stop attending a meeting? Could you achieve the task in a different way, without the meeting? Does the meeting need to happen at all?

Depending on your level of seniority, this may be one you will have to discuss with your manager before you simply stop attending meetings. But if you can make a genuine case that your presence for an hour (or more) isn't adding anything and you can contribute just as well by reading the minutes afterwards, then you have the opportunity to work during that time on something that does benefit the company or is related to your core role.

David Allen suggests there are five reasons for holding a meeting, and that it's critical everyone in the meeting is on the same page on which of these your meeting is trying to achieve.

1. To give information
2. To get information
3. To develop options
4. To make decisions
5. Warm, magical human contact

Consider the next three meeting appointments in your diary. Write the meeting subject of each opposite, then write the one (or more) of David Allen's "five reasons for holding a meeting" that match with each of the three meetings.

1.

_____

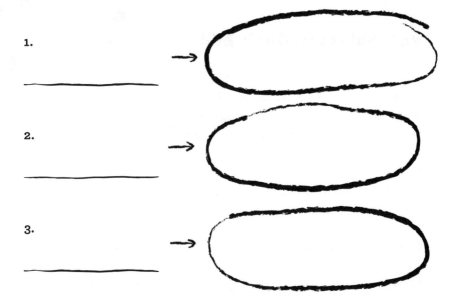

2.

_____

3.

_____

Are you adding anything personally to these meetings that couldn't
be achieved outside the meetings more quickly?

— — — — — — — — — — —

Can the purpose of any of the three meetings be achieved in a
different way, without holding the meeting?

— — — — — — — — — — —

Talk to the relevant people and see if there is at least one meeting
that you could stop attending.

#47 Subtract, Don't Add

Many of us have a tendency to add things to our to-do lists, e.g. "I should do more development around leadership". However, we don't always consider the idea of subtracting things, which can make our projects or our work life both more focused and, in many cases, more effective.

Consider, is there anything you have on your to-do list that's not going to add a lot of usefulness or value? Is there something that's been on there for weeks, but you're never going to get round to completing?

Complete the sentence:

I can remove _ _ _ _ _ _ _ _ _ _ _ _ from my to-do list.

What would the impact of this be?

_____

_____

_____

_____

_____

_____

_____

#48 Limit the Scope

To be productive, we also need to make sure we're focusing our energy on the right activities, and avoid "scope creep" – that is, when the original task keeps growing, because either you or others are adding unnecessary activities, while keeping the same deadline, which can make it an impossible task.

We can ensure this doesn't happen by agreeing a list of "deliverables" with whoever delegates a piece of work to us – whether it's our manager or a client. Once delivered to the other person, these will show the project is finished.

For most of us, if we communicate well with the other people involved and agree at the start what is needed, then when we're done, we can point back to the pre-determined list and show that we've delivered what was agreed.

We need to watch out for people adding unnecessary or extra deliverables after the project has started, and to manage and document if any changes are asked for. We also need to communicate the impact of that change – whether it's more time, money or resources that might be needed.

Think about one of your projects or tasks. How will you know it is finished? What do you need to "deliver" to your manager or client to show you have completed the task or project?

_____

_____

How will you manage when someone asks you for something extra on top of what has been agreed?

_____

_____

#49 Doing Time versus Deciding Time

One trap we often fall into is trying to do both "deciding" activities and "doing" activities in the same session. This means we can be trying to work on an activity without being sure what we're supposed to do next, and this can also be a big cause of procrastination.

We are much more likely to be successful if we split up "deciding" time and "doing" time, so that the decisions on what to do next have been separated from the time we sit down at our desk ready to get on with the activity.

For example, if I know I need to prepare a lesson plan as a teacher, before I start "doing" the lesson plan, I need to do some "deciding" – i.e. what the topic is, what my structure looks like, how will I know when it's ready.

Write down one of the larger tasks you are working on at the moment.

_____

_____

_____

What are the next three actions you need to take to complete this task? (You are "deciding" here.) When will you do these actions? (Schedule in your "doing" time.)

1.

When will you do this?

2.

When will you do this?

3.

When will you do this?

#50 Set Goals You Can Actually Achieve

One challenge with a lot of the goals we set is that they are "fluffy". By that, I mean they have a big, vague idea at the end, without clarity on how to achieve it.

SMART (see below) is a well-known acronym to remind us how to set goals that are achievable. Clarifying how we will achieve our goals enhances our work wellness by removing the stress of being weighed down by a goal we don't really know how to accomplish, and helps stop us procrastinating.

Making a goal SMART is linked to **#49 Doing Time versus Deciding Time** – it means we are clearly using our deciding time to make the goal SMART and can focus on the doing time later.

SMART goals are:

Specific: Set narrow, clear goals with detail (for example, consider who, what, where)

Measurable: Set goals that are trackable rather than vague so you are clear when the goal has been achieved

Attainable: Set goals that are challenging but possible, and know the steps you will take to achieve them

Relevant: Set goals that are useful to what you want to achieve, and in line with your values and your job role

Time-bound: Set goals with a deadline

An example of an un-SMART goal would be: "I will grow the organization's social media presence."

An example of a SMART goal would be: "I will increase the organization's social media followers on Instagram and Facebook by 5 per cent by the end of June. I will do this through the use of Facebook and Instagram advertising."

Pick a goal you want to achieve, and redefine it as a SMART goal.

ORIGINAL GOAL

_____

_____

SMART GOAL

_____

_____

_____

_____

_____

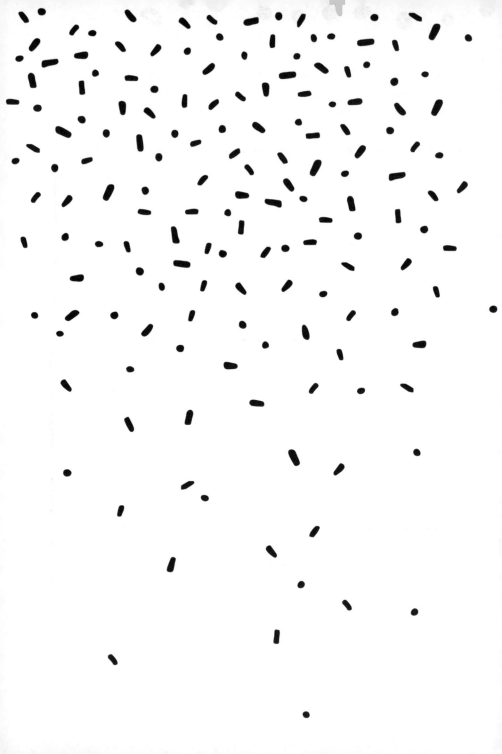

CHAPTER 6

Breaks

Breaks

The idea that taking a break will support your work wellness shouldn't be a shocking. However, 55 per cent of Americans and 62 per cent of UK workers don't use all their vacation days, which means they are essentially providing free labour on those days to their employers.

And while you'd think, if you're self-employed, you could take a break at any time, as you're not entitled to holiday pay and will take a financial hit for every day you don't work, the pressure to keep grinding away can be intense.

However, research conducted on productivity suggests that working more hours doesn't automatically lead to a higher output. Indeed, after a 50-hour week, productivity falls steeply, whereas a 35–40-hour week is most correlated with happiness.

In addition, when we work long hours, our sleep usually takes a hit. This causes a decline in our creativity and problem solving. Lack of sleep is especially detrimental for knowledge workers, as the less sleep you have, the more error-prone you are likely to be, and the more you limit your ability to organize and process information and perform at your optimum level.

When we consider the fact that we are likely to be more productive, not less, if our brain gets time away from the business of the day-to-day grind, taking breaks becomes a critical part of creating the conditions for our best work self.

What you will find in this chapter

In this chapter we are reminded, firstly, to **#51 Use Breaks**, then we will look at the longer term and think about the need to **#52 Take Holidays**. We will also consider a third way to take breaks with **#53 Take a Break From a Specific Task**.

Once we've lined up the types of breaks we can take, we will start thinking about how you might *use* those breaks. **#54 20/20/20** reminds us of the importance of eye health, while **#55 Don't Eat at Your Desk** and **#56 Eat Mindfully** consider how and where you consume food on your breaks, and what you can do to make sure your eating supports your work vitality. Other ways to use breaks include **#57 Naps** and **#58 Walking Meetings**.

We finish the section by thinking about how to bring more **#59 Awe and Wonder** to your day, along with the benefits when you **#60 Incorporate Playfulness in Breaks**.

#51 Use Breaks

You need time to recharge. Taking the breaks you are legally allowed or, if you're self-employed, finding time for yourself during your day (without your eyes being glued to your phone), will have multiple benefits.

If you can take your break outside, great; if you can find some nature to spend it in, brilliant. Otherwise, while perhaps less inspiring, walking up and down the stairs or around the car park will still get you a change of scene and some movement.

What do your breaks look like at work?

If you work for a company, do you have to take them at particular times? Do you know what you are entitled to from a legal perspective? Do you know what the "company culture norm" is for breaks?

If you're self-employed, do you take breaks? How do you recharge during your day? What break time could you include in your regular day to give yourself some time away from technology?

How could you use your breaks across a day to give you more time away from the screen, to break up your work and to give you some fresh air, exercise or time to eat something away from your desk?

#52 Take Holidays

There are plenty of benefits to taking annual leave: the opportunity to connect with others, explore new places or interests, manage your stress levels by relaxing, catch up on a sleep debt and more.

If you're self-employed, at the start of the year commit to taking a certain number of days off as holiday. If you're unsure about how many you should have, you can use the time organizations give their workers as a starting point.

The UK and US approach holiday time differently. In the UK, employees who work five or more days a week are entitled to 28 days of paid leave including bank holidays. In the US, workers are not entitled to a single day as statutory, although, on average, US workers receive 10 days of paid holiday each year. So, decide how many days you want to give yourself between 10 and 28 days.

Review your annual leave allowance or decide how many days you want to give yourself per year if you're self-employed.

How many days off do you currently have planned into your diary?

How many days do you still need to schedule?

Put a reminder in your diary once a month to repeat this activity, changing the numbers (how many days you are allowed, how many are planned, how many you have left) each month. This will stop you "forgetting" to schedule it in.

Colour in the star when you're done!

#53 Take a Break From a Specific Task

Sometimes, doing something different for a period can act as a "break" for the mind. Idea **#43 Use Pomodoros** is one example of this. As discussed earlier, you need to find what works for you in terms of blocks of time, but I find switching between two activities – something more intense for the longer blocks and something less intense, like admin, for the shorter blocks – can work well.

This isn't about switching from task to task aimlessly, as that's likely to cause distraction, and it's also not about "multitasking". This is about concentrating on one activity, then doing another, then going back to the first in a deliberate fashion to refresh you.

Look at your tasks for the day. Are there two tasks, one more intense, one less so, that you could schedule in this way? Block out an hour to experiment with this.

Write the schedule and the tasks opposite.

Then come back here and consider: how did it go?

Time schedued	Task
15 minutes	work on report
5 minutes	answer emails
15 minutes	work on report
5 minutes	answer emails
10 minutes	break

#54 20/20/20

Our eyes haven't evolved to focus on objects at such a short distance for such long periods, as we do when we focus on our screens. When we don't give our eyes a break, we can cause ourselves eye strain or other eye problems – research suggests almost half of office workers experience these at some time.

To avoid such problems, clinical optometrists suggest the 20/20/20 rule – for every 20 minutes of close-up work, look at something 20m (65½ft) away for at least 20 seconds. If you're in a small space, simply look out of a window.

Set an alarm to remind you to 20/20/20 – you can also use every third of these to #23 Get Up and Move!

Look out of your window now and draw what you see.

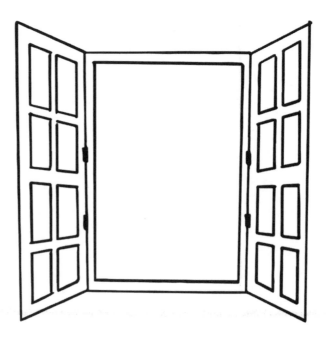

#55 Don't Eat at Your Desk

If you carried out idea **#9 Wipe Down Your Technology**, you might have been a little horrified when you saw the crumbs and other dirt that had lodged in your keyboard. Eating at our desk, while very common, is suboptimal for hygiene, digestion and **#24 Thresholding**.

If we don't step away from our desk to eat somewhere else, then the line between our work and everything else is blurred further. We need the downtime for our busy brains to rest for a bit between activities.

Eat somewhere other than at your desk this week:

- If you're working in a café, change tables and shut your laptop.

- If you're working at home, go to the kitchen or another place in the house.

- If you're working in an office, go outside or to the cafeteria or break room.

How did you feel taking this eating break?

Can you commit to doing this at least 80 per cent of the time for your snacks and meals from now on?

#56 Eat Mindfully

When you do eat (remembering **#55 Don't Eat at Your Desk**), take your time. Chew each bite thoroughly, and enjoy the food. Take this opportunity to be mindful and grateful that you have access to nourishment.

Eating more mindfully helps optimize digestive function, while enhancing self-acceptance, mind-body-food awareness and overall wellness.

You don't have to linger for hours but, at the very least, *notice* that you're eating and really look at the food in front of you.

For at least one meal or snack a day this week, eat mindfully.

Journal on how it felt different from the way you usually approach your food at work and what thoughts arose.

#57 Naps

This one might be a bit more challenging, but studies indicate that there can be health benefits to a short nap. This is likely one where those who work at home are in a better position to experiment with the idea, but it may also be possible to use your car to take a quick nap in.

In some Asian countries, it's very normal to nap at your desk during breaks, but it's less likely to be welcomed in western cultures, so take this into consideration. Your commute can also be a time to nap (assuming you're not in charge of the vehicle and, if you're using public transport, you might want to set an alarm so you don't miss your stop!). An alternative is a quick nap as soon as you come home from work to refresh yourself before your evening starts – and there's always the rest room…!

Naps of 10 to 20 minutes seem to work best, up to a maximum of 30 minutes. Always set an alarm, and one top tip is to drink a coffee beforehand so the caffeine has a chance to get working just as you wake up. You could even sit and mindfully take two minutes with your eyes closed to offer you a mini nap break and a sense of pressing pause.

Make a plan for how and when you could fit power naps into your daily schedule this week.

WHEN	HOW

#58 Walking Meetings

One good way of changing things up and giving yourself a break while also "being productive" can be to schedule some walking meetings. This tends to work best when it's a one-to-one meeting where you're having a catch up – probably sharing information or giving information, as well as some warm, magical human contact. If you need to take notes, it can be more challenging, but this can be managed by bringing a notepad and stopping on a park bench every 20 minutes or so, or dictating notes into your phone.

It's surprising that we are often prepared to share more or be more vulnerable when we're walking along side by side than when we're sitting opposite each other making direct eye contact. It can also make it easier to share feedback.

Who in your meeting schedule would be both appropriate and willing to experiment with you by doing a walking meeting?

Draft an email here to ask them the next time you have a meeting together in the diary.

When you've had the meeting, come back here and journal on:

What were the differences between this meeting and your regular meetings?

How did it feel?

What worked well?

What didn't work?

What do you need to change next time?

#59 Awe and Wonder

It's also worth thinking about how you spend your breaks, and the next two ideas consider that. One thing that has been shown to help us in a myriad of ways, but particularly around finding perspective, is thinking about something that creates a sense of awe and wonder in you. Of course, it's harder to climb a mountain or catch a rainbow in person while you're at work, but you could watch a video or look at a picture or even read a description in a book. Examples include natural wonders like the Grand Canyon or feats of construction like Angkor Wat. Nature provides a lot of opportunity for this.

However, don't think that if you're working in a town or city you can't find moments of awe and wonder. Look for trees, birds, interesting architecture – the best tip here is to look up!

What creates a sense of awe and wonder in you?

_____

_____

Name three ways that you could echo this feeling while at work:

1.

2.

3.

#60 Incorporate Playfulness in Breaks

Playfulness has been shown to support creativity and is another way of spending a break doing something that can nurture you. Your environment is going to make a big difference when it comes to finding ways to incorporate play in your breaks, of course, but it's a vast area of opportunity, as play can take many forms. Play itself can be any leisure activity (physical or mental) that is undertaken purely for enjoyment and amusement without other objectives. Examples include:

- Ritual play – chess, board games or any sport with set rules
- Rough and tumble play – physical games like dodgeball
- Imaginative play – colouring, acting, storytelling
- Body play – messing around with gravity, through yoga, hiking or even jumping on a mini-trampoline
- Object play – playing with Lego, Jenga or designing and building something physical

Clearly some of these are harder than others in the workplace – but your set-up – and your imagination – are the only limits.

Name five ways you could include some play into your work breaks this week:

1. _____

2. _____

3. _____

4. _____

5. _____

CHAPTER 7

Time Management

Time Management

In some ways, managing our time effectively is at the heart of our ability to flourish at work. If we can plan out the time we have available and use it in the best way possible, balancing breaks and work, taking time to nourish ourselves and time to be productive, we are much more likely to blossom and grow. This also includes protecting and prioritizing our time, as well as ensuring we don't "waste" it by procrastinating or spending it on activities that don't move us forward in some way or **#16 Use Your Values** and "why" (**#12 Name Your Work Why**).

However, we all need downtime, and managing your time doesn't mean being on the go and filling every minute of your day. It means ensuring you include recharging time, breaks, social time and all the different aspects that this book shares to help you be your best self at work. Developing the ability to make decisions and control how you spend your time will help you with all the other areas of work wellness, so it's really worth focusing your attention on.

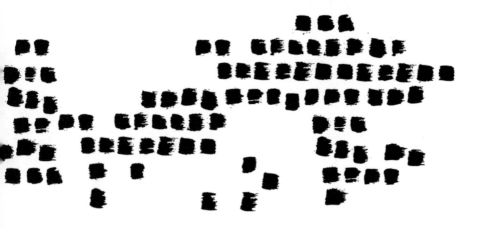

What you can find in this chapter

In this chapter, we'll start by exploring how to **#61 Time Track**, which will help support you to **#62 Plan – Realistically** and ensure you have a **#63 Safety Margins** for when tasks overrun unexpectedly.

Once you have a good handle on how you spend your time, you will be more empowered to **#64 Say No** appropriately.

We'll work on getting things done more quickly in **#65 Cut 5 per cent**, using the **#66 Two-Minute Rule** and making sure we **#67 Don't "Touch" Something More Than Three Times**.

Next we'll step back and consider **#68 The Right Time** in your day to plan different types of activity to do your best work, as well as experimenting with giving all your attention to **#69 A Single Task**.

Finally, you'll **#70 Get an Accountability Partner** to make sure you get things done on time, using the external support to stick to your commitments.

#61 Time Track

One mistake many of us make when planning out our time is to look at the eight-hour work day and plan tasks to fill it completely.

However, an eight-hour day is not eight hours of productive time. We take breaks, we get interrupted, the situation changes, it's hard to predict how much time something will take exactly, etc. If you try to schedule eight full hours in your day, you will always be behind, and feeling behind is not helpful for work wellness!

You can explore this by time tracking, where you look in detail at what you actually do each day.

For example, in this day, the person planned to spend 8 hours on Project X - but only managed 4 hours and 40 minutes:

09.00 – Come in, sit down greet others [social – 15 mins]
09.15 – Check emails, respond [admin – 30 mins]
09.45 – Work on Project X [productive time – 45 mins]
10.30 – Get coffee, chat to Brian about his new project [social – 10 mins]
10.40 – Work on Project X [productive time – 50 mins]
11.30 – Team meeting [team time – 60 mins]
12.30 – Lunch [break – 45 mins]
13.15 – Check emails, realize emergency on Project Y [admin – 15 mins]
13.30 – Work on Project Y [productive time, unplanned – 30 mins]
14.00 – Work on Project X [productive time – 45 mins]
14.45 – Interrupted by colleague who needed help [team time – 30 mins]
15.15 – Work on Project X [productive time – 15 mins]
15.30 – Get a drink [break – 10 mins]
15.40 – Work on Project X [productive time – 65 mins]
16.45 – Manager needs something [team time – 15 mins]
17.00 – Work on Project X [productive time – 60 mins]
18.00 – Home

Track what you spend your time on for one day this week and see what you actually do, so you can get an idea of what you can realistically achieve in the time you have available.

Time	Activity	Time category (productive, team, etc.)

#62 Plan – Realistically

After you have explored **#61 Time Track**, you are likely to have a range
of, say, four to six hours of productive time in a day, and you can now plan
more realistically. At the very least, it will tell you when you might need to
do overtime!

Pick a day next week and plan it out here.

Planned activity	What actually happened

Once you have lived the day, write next to your plan what actually
happened in a different coloured pen.

Is your planning getting more realistic? What else could you do to
tweak it more effectively?

#63 Safety Margins

The exercises in ideas **#61 Time Track** and **#62 Plan – Realistically**
probably showed you that the amount of time tasks will take can be
harder to predict than you think, and that it takes experience to refine
your understanding of what is realistic when planning. But even when
you think you have a good handle on the time it takes to do a task, you
need to add in a safety margin, for unexpected interruptions or risks.

You will need to play with your safety margin – 10 per cent or 20 per cent
extra time is typical – to balance what you need to get done, the extra hours
you might work and realism. Remember: it's far better to promise work
delivered at a later date and then deliver early than the other way round.

If nothing extra then comes up, great! You can use that safety margin time
for whatever works. However, if an emergency or crisis does happen, you're
not suddenly working 10 per cent overtime or finding yourself 10 per cent
behind on one of the other things you had planned to do that day.

**Which of my activities, days or tasks would most benefit from a
safety margin?**

_____

Where and how can I add this in?

_____

Who (if anyone) do I need to talk to about adding this in?

_____

What might be the consequences of adding it in?

_____

_____

#64 Say No

With a more realistic perspective on your day, it's easier to understand what you can – and can't – say yes to. While you might sometimes choose to be strategic and take on extra work because of a new project, there are also going to be times when you're going to have to say no. It is not possible to do everything! Saying no is rarely easy, but remember the line "every time you say yes to something, you say no to something else". Given that, isn't it better to be in charge of what you're saying no to?

Here are some suggestions on how to say no in different ways when your schedule is already overfull for the week.

To your manager: *Right now, I have a full week doing X, Y and Z. I could do this if I postpone something for X time. What is your suggestion on the best way forward here?*

To a colleague who wants you to help them: *I'm really busy at the moment, but I think [insert name here] might be able to help you with that.*

To a colleague who wants you to take on something new: *I don't have time in the schedule this week, but I'd love to help you on [insert date here]. Let me know if you still need me then.*

To someone who wants to get coffee and "pick your brains": *I appreciate the thought, but my time is already maxed out at the moment. However, the resource [insert resource name] addresses this topic really well, so why don't you take a look at that and ping me with any questions that come up?*

It can also help if you focus on your "why" (**#12 Name Your Work Why**) or **#16 Use Your Values**. Alternatively, you could simply list your top three priorities at work at the moment, and if something comes up that doesn't connect with these, it might not be the right project or task for you, and you can share that with the person asking.

Write two scripts for the most common things you are asked to do that you want to say no to in future. Practise reading them aloud so they become graceful and natural.

Script 1

_____

_____

_____

_____

_____

Script 2

_____

_____

_____

_____

_____

#65 Cut 5 per cent

Counterintuitively, the next activity suggests you trim time from your most common tasks, to build the muscle of working through information quickly and accurately. As you progress to become more senior in organizations, you will need to deal with more information and to do so more quickly.

It's a challenging muscle to build, but one small experiment you can try is to take a typical task – one which you already know will take you a given amount of time – like checking your emails in the morning. If it typically takes you an hour to do this, set a timer for 57 minutes (5 per cent less time) instead, and aim to work through your emails just a little bit more quickly. After a week, try for 54 minutes (10 per cent less time than the original 60 minutes).

Pick a task you do regularly, at least a few times a week.

— —   — —   — —   — —   — —   —

Time yourself for a week on that task. What is the average time it takes you?

— — —   — — — —   — — — —

Remove small increments of time until you've found a realistic amount of time to aim for.

How did this feel?

— —   — —   — —   — —   — —   —

— —   — —   — —   — —   — —   —

#66 Two-Minute Rule

This is one of my favourite tools, and it's easy enough – essentially, if you know a task is only going to take you two minutes or less, DO IT NOW; don't wait till later.

Examples might include:

- Opening the post
- Dealing with an email
- Washing up a coffee cup
- Making a call
- Unsubscribing from a mailing list

List three things that would have taken you two minutes or less that you didn't do the first time they came up, and think about why you didn't complete each one immediately.

Two-minute tasks	Why didn't you do it immediately?
1.	
2.	
3.	

Is there any reason why in the future you couldn't do any of these tasks in two minutes next time?

If not, look out for these tasks as they come up this week, and make sure you do them in two minutes.

#67 Don't "Touch" Something More Than Three Times

When we leave something in our inbox, or have a task that's waiting for us, it can drag at our attention, creating a psychic weight far more than if we just got it off our plate. This idea suggests you make a rule not to "touch" (or interact) with something more than three times before it's done.

What this might mean to you is, instead of reading an email in your inbox 20 times and feeling guilty, you do something with it before you get to the third time. For example:

1. Read an email. Make a note of the activities it requires and put them on your list. File the email in an "ongoing" file. Do the activities.

2. Come back to the email and reply to say it's dealt with. Move the email to wherever you keep "dealt with" emails.

Look at your physical desk, computer desktop and email. Is there anything on, or in, any of them that requires action?

Write down opposite the items and the actions they require (note: this is a type of "deciding" time as per idea #49 Doing Time versus Deciding Time; you're not aiming to do the actions, just to decide what's next).

File the appropriate documents electronically or in a physical folder, so you're not looking at them while you're not taking action. You can create "action" or "ongoing" or some such folders if you need a holding file, but don't put anything in these folders without having the associated action written down somewhere or they become their own special black holes!

Item	Next Actions

#68 The Right Time

Different tasks need different energy levels or focus and concentration from us. Research suggests we are likely to use our time better if we schedule the task to match the energy level we have at that time, as this and our cognitive abilities fluctuate over a day.

Let's look at an example. While most of us want to start with something easy when we begin our office day, like email and admin, the research suggests we have more energy, positivity and motivation in the morning versus the afternoon, so starting on a more difficult task might reap greater benefits than starting with something easy, which you could leave till your afternoon "trough".

Get to know your energy levels.

When during the day do you feel most energized?

....

When do you experience a "trough" or drop in energy?

....

When does your energy return?

....

Be sensitive to which activities in the day best fit your energy levels. Make a list of each so that, wherever possible, you can pick your tasks to suit your current level.

#69 A Single Task

Doing one thing at a time. Such a simple idea – yet how many of us actually manage it? Rather than helping us do more, multitasking actually diminishes our performance. Doing one activity at a time, with all our attention and focus, is likely to reduce the time the activity takes and get a better-quality outcome. This exercise helps you practise, and I would suggest combining it with **#42 Pull the Plug** and **#43 Use Pomodoros** to get the most from it.

Pick any activity, from making your morning drink to working on a report.

Remove any distractions from your environment (put your phone on silent, close other windows, etc.).

For five minutes (use a timer!) focus only on the task you have chosen.

Repeatedly bring your attention back to the task if it wanders.

Use the appropriate senses to engage with the task.

How did it feel to single-task?

_____

_____

What will you practise on next?

_____

_____

#70 Get an Accountability Partner

Sharing with another person that you have committed to a certain action by a certain time is likely to help you get the task done.

Making a public or semi-public commitment in this way makes us feel more obliged to meet the expectations we have set, as we don't want to let that person down by not being true to the commitment we have made.

Share with a friend or colleague that you'd like them to be an accountability partner for you.

Tell them you will give them updates on the task at whatever interval works for you (for example, on a smaller project it might be daily; on a bigger project it might be weekly).

Write down the friend/colleague's name and tick each time you check in with them.

Name

_____

Check in date

_____ ☐

_____ ☐

_____ ☐

_____ ☐

Once the task or activity is complete, journal below about the difference it made having an accountability partner.

_____

_____

_____

_____

_____

_____

_____

_____

CHAPTER 8

Work Relationships

Work Relationships

Relationships are critical at work, where we are surrounded by a network of people, some of whom we may end up interacting and spending time with more than our friends or families. Even if we are self-employed working alone at home, we are likely to have clients, suppliers and other people in our network.

Relationships with co-workers have been identified as one of the top drivers of employee engagement and also have a positive effect on teamwork, productivity, satisfaction and morale.

Humans have a strong desire to be connected with others, and interpersonal relationships have a huge impact on our wellness both inside and outside work.

So there are plenty of reasons to concentrate energy and time on the relationships we have with those we work with. We can think about these relationships in terms of "interaction" (how often we communicate or associate with others) and "relatedness" (the amount we have in common).

Thus, one way to improve our relationships at work is to take more opportunities for interaction and use them to build relatedness.

What you will find in this chapter

In this chapter you will first consider **#71 What is Your Personal Brand**, a reflection on how you would like to be seen by others in the workplace.

You'll consider **#72 Who Do You Want to Be Around?**, and then the reverse – **#73 Do People Want to Be Around You?**

You'll think about tactics to support your work relationships through opportunities to **#74 Offer Help** and **#75 Ask for Help**. You can also **#76 Offer Feedback** to help others improve.

#77 Say Thank You is a simple but often neglected concept. More challenging but equally important is to build loyalty and trust when you **#78 Take Responsibility**.

In an unusual idea, you can build relationships when you **#79 Gossip Appropriately**.

Finally, remember to **#80 Schedule Time for Work Relationships**, when you can put all the ideas into practice.

#71 What is Your Personal Brand?

Just as organizations have a brand, we each have aspects that make us distinct from those around us – our personal brand. A personal brand at work could include everything from the way you dress to how you interact with others to your values to anything others are likely to associate with you.

Thinking about our brand and what we want it to be helps us to align our behaviours with it, and provides another way to guide us in the direction of the best version of ourselves in the way we interact with others at work.

Use visuals (draw, or cut out and stick pictures in), words or sentences to represent what you would like your personal brand to be.

For example, write words that you would like others to associate with you (clever, creative, well-dressed, organized, funny, reliable, etc.).

What one action can you take today to show this personal brand to others?

#72 Who Do You Want to Be Around?

We rarely choose the people we work with, whether they are colleagues, suppliers, clients or anyone else we interact with for work. But just as relationships are critical in our home life, they can make a big difference at work too. A key predictor of whether you feel engaged with your work is if you feel you have a "good friend" you can talk to in the work sphere.

Write the names of anyone you interact with for work, putting those who you feel closest to nearer to the central "me" circle, and those you feel less of a connection with further away from it.

Place a "+" by anyone you would like to spend more time with

Place a "−" by anyone you would like to spend less time with

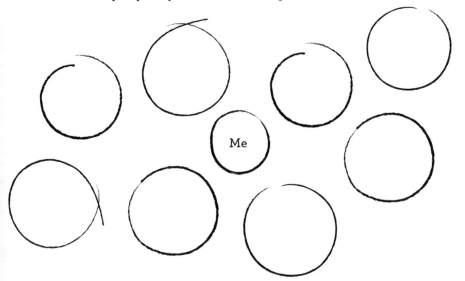

What action can you take to make one of these changes happen?

#73 Do People Want to Be Around You?

It's not just about your needs and who you want to be friends with at work;
you also need to consider if you are a good friend to your colleagues, or at
least the ones you want to be close to.

What do you feel are the five most important qualities of a friend,
particularly in the work context?

1. _____ __ _____ __ ___ __
2. _____ _____ ___
3. _____ __ _____ __ _____ __ __
4. _____ _____ ____
5. _____ __ _____ __ _____ ___ __

Pick someone you would like to build a closer relationship with,
then choose one of the above qualities and consider how you could
demonstrate more of this to your friend over the next week.

#74 Offer Help

One great way to build relationships at work, as well as boost your own morale, is to offer your support. This can come in many guises, depending on your strengths and your availability – from lending a listening ear over coffee to reviewing a piece of someone's work to offering other freelancers support.

Fill in the following:

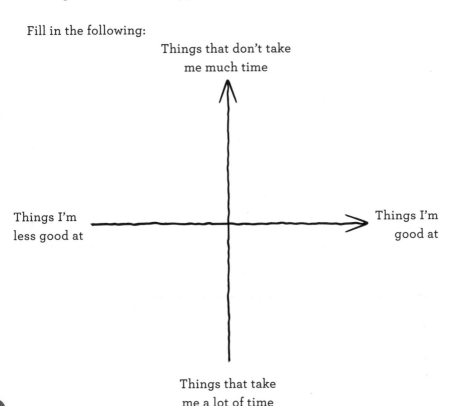

Things that don't take
me much time

Things I'm
less good at

Things I'm
good at

Things that take
me a lot of time

Pick something from the top right – "things I'm good at/things that don't take me much time", then think of a person who might benefit and enjoy your support in this area, and gently sound them out to see if it might be welcomed.

#75 Ask for Help

Perhaps surprisingly, asking for help also has benefits in terms of
relationships. The person who is being asked gets a self-esteem boost,
and research shows they are likely to want to help you even more in the
future. There's even evidence that asking for a favour can turn enemies
into friends! Many of us are more comfortable giving help than getting
it, however, so we need to work the muscle.

What's the most challenging issue facing you at work right now?

What kind of help would you benefit from?

Who might be able to provide that help?

Draft a script or email asking them for that help:

Now go ask them!

#76 Offer Feedback

Getting into the practice of giving others feedback – both constructive and positive – about their work has many benefits. It can be a way of ensuring your positive/negative ratio (**#11 One Positive Interaction a Day**) stays at at least 5:1, and by feeding back regularly, not just when you have criticism, people are more likely to welcome your less positive feedback when you do want to share it.

In turn, they're also more likely to be comfortable giving you feedback, which will help you with your development. Identifying others' development areas and strengths will help you with your own work wellness as you get more comfortable understanding behaviour. This idea also combines nicely with the Development and Growth chapter.

Tips:

- Make your feedback about their actions, not about them as a person
- Give context – explain the impact of their actions
- Make it timely – don't leave it a long time between the actions and the feedback
- Keep it relatively short
- Include more positives than negatives

Example: Thanks so much for working with me on the X project. I really appreciated your support, timeliness and your attention to detail. I think you did a great job working with our supplier, who I know is fairly demanding. One thing that might be helpful on future projects would be to connect more frequently with colleagues to update them on the project – weekly updates rather than unplanned updates would ensure everyone's on the same page. Thanks again for all your work, and I look forward to working with you again in the future.

Pick a person you've worked with in the last month and, remembering the tips above, write down a) what they did well and b) what they could have done differently.

Person:

What they did well:

What they could have done differently:

This is practice; you don't need to give them this feedback unless you want to, but look out for opportunities to offer feedback in the future.

#77 Say Thank You

This one may be easy, but it's also easily forgotten. Showing gratitude is another practice that benefits both giver and receiver, and the relationship between you both.

When you say thank you, be specific. So, rather than "Thanks for your help", say, "Thanks for your help with the XX presentation. I appreciated you sending me such detailed feedback on my draft so quickly, and it really improved the quality of the final piece of work."

Here you've said:

- What you're saying thank you for
- What they did that helped you
- The impact it had

Craft a thank you here to a work colleague, then share it with the relevant person.

Thank you for....

#78 Take Responsibility

The respect, loyalty and support of others in the workplace can make a huge difference to our work wellness – but we have to earn them by first showing these qualities to those we work with. The key to this is stepping up and taking responsibility for our mistakes (**#31 How to Rectify a Mistake: Acknowledge it** and **#32 How to Rectify a Mistake: Make it Right**) and not publicly sacrificing someone else for your own gain.

Think of a time in your career where someone else let you take responsibility for their mistake.

_____

_____

What happened?

_____

_____

What was the impact of their actions on your relationship?

_____

_____

Now consider: If you were in their situation, what would you do differently?

_____

_____

#79 Gossip Appropriately

Gossip is often considered a bad thing, but when we think about it as sharing information about others when they are not there, it can be either positive, neutral or negative.

In fact, talking about people is a big part of everyone's lives (female *and* male!), and helps us gain social information in big networks of people, as well as allowing us to navigate complex social behaviours. There's also a type of more "negative" gossip, used to warn others about someone's untrustworthiness or mean behaviour, called "prosocial gossip". This latter type deters selfishness and promotes cooperation in others by ensuring their reputation is potentially damaged if they behave badly.

Engaging in "helpful gossip" (about things that are true and positive, neutral or prosocial) can create intimacy through shared feelings and experiences, which can stave off loneliness, and facilitate bonding and closeness.

Examples of gossip:

Did you know Raj Shetty has been made Head of the Research Department? (Neutral)

Chioma Olaleye drove her project hard but delivered it on time and under budget. (Positive)

Watch out for Hugh Menthel - he has a tendency to take credit for projects from other people. (Prosocial)

Write down either a positive/neutral/prosocial piece of gossip here:

#80 Schedule Time for Work Relationships

It can be hard to find time for work relationships in a world where we're busy, but investing in the network of relationships at work is likely to pay you back both personally and professionally. This means scoping out a bit of time to nurture the social side of work – and expanding your social network in a gentle way to do this. Combine with **#74 Offer Help** and **#75 Ask for Help** for even more benefits.

Name two people at work you are already friendly with who you'd like to catch up with.

1.

2.

Identify one person at work who you'd like to get to know better, and consider how and when you might do this.

Name

Method

Scheduled for

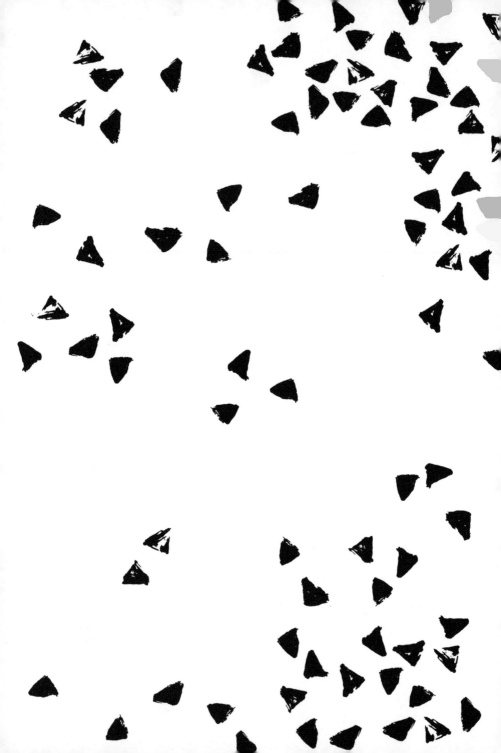

CHAPTER 9

Development and Growth

Development and Growth

Development and growth are a particular passion of mine, both as an individual and work psychologist. In many ways all the ideas in this book (as well as my previous book, *This Is For You*) are about personal and professional growth, and are designed to support you in becoming the best version of you. This chapter focuses more on professional growth, in terms of knowledge, skills, behaviours and other attributes.

Sometimes at work people develop themselves until they get to a certain position, at which point they decide they're "done" and stop putting in the effort. However, this is very different from athletes or musicians, for example, who never stop practising and working on their technique. Why should it be different for us in our professional lives? We can *always* grow further as a professional, as a person, as a work colleague, as a manager and in any of the other roles we take on at work.

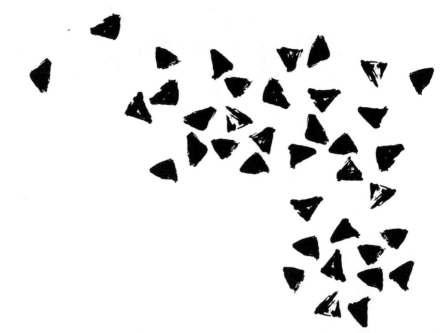

What you will find in this chapter

In this chapter you'll start by considering the big picture, giving yourself a goal to aim at by outlining your #**81 Perfect Work Day**.

Then you'll look at the gap between where you are now and that ideal picture, first as you **#82 Assess Your Own Development Needs** and then when you **#83 Get to Know What You Need to Develop**. To keep spirits high during this period of reflection, we'll **#84 Keep a Success File**.

Next you'll **#85 Decide Your Next Steps**, and then **#86 Break it Down** into manageable steps, while you **#87 Keep a Development Journal** to stay on track and record progress.

You'll leverage your work friendships to **#88 Find a Peer Mentor or Coach**, while you learn by teaching and **#89 Share Knowledge**.

Finally, you'll **#90 Grow Your Ability to Handle Emotions** – an under-considered area at work, but one which can make a big difference to the way you interact with others in the workplace.

#81 Perfect Work Day

Start with the big picture, so you have context for what you want to develop and grow in yourself.

Take some time to visualize what your ideal work day looks like.

- What time would it start?
- What location would you work from?
- What tasks would it involve?
- Which people would you see?
- When would it end?
- What skills or qualities do you need to develop to be able to live this sort of work day?

Describe your perfect work day using the questions above as your starting point:

#82 Assess Your Own Development Needs

Before you start to invest time developing anything, you first need to take stock of what you feel you bring to your role and the organization you work for in terms of behaviours, skills, knowledge, competencies, abilities, personality traits and anything else that may be relevant.

Take 15 minutes to complete the following questions.

What do I do well (i.e. what are my strengths) and what can I develop (i.e. what are my weaknesses)?

Mark the top three strengths you want to build on with a *, as well as the top three development areas you want to focus on.

#83 Get to Know What You Need to Develop

Reality-check your self-assessment by getting feedback on your performance from others with a couple of simple questions:

- "What do I do well?"
- "What can I do differently?"

Ask by email, as it is less confrontational and won't put them on the spot, but give them a deadline of a week so there is some urgency. You could start the email by saying something like this:

As part of a development exercise I am doing, I hope you won't mind if I ask you to share your thoughts on two questions. It would help me if you can be honest. Thanks so much for your time.

Remember to always say thank you, whatever the feedback! Receiving feedback gracefully is your part of this activity.

Make a list of 3–10 people who see you in a variety of contexts (for example, your boss, teammates, customers, subordinates, suppliers) who you could ask for feedback on your performance in the past six months.

☐   ☐

☐   ☐

☐   ☐

☐   ☐

☐   ☐

#84 Keep a Success File

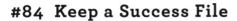

For moments when you're feeling low and need a little positivity to cheer you up, keeping a list of your successes at work can prove highly beneficial. This file can also be very useful when you are putting together information for performance reviews, a case for promotion, a CV or preparing for interviews.

In your success file, write down things that went well – anything from a compliment from a colleague – to winning a new project to achieving the highest sales numbers in your company for the year. The key is to make keeping this file up to date as easy as you possibly can.

Choose a method and place for keeping your success file.

How often will you update it?

What can you put in your success file now?

#85 Decide Your Next Steps

Even if we're happy with the status quo and not seeking to make our business bigger or get promoted, it can help us focus if we have a goal that allows us to get closer to our perfect work day. The goal might be maintaining or improving our appraisal rating, finishing a project with good feedback from our customer or hitting our target – whatever feels relevant to you. Remember: increasing your work wellness and enjoying your work more can be goals too!

Making the goal specific and knowing how you will achieve it (using the principles in **#50 Set Goals You Can Actually Achieve**) will help you to plot a clear path.

What are your current work goals?

_____

_____

What do you need to do to achieve them?

_____

_____

What strengths can you use?

_____

_____

What skills do you need to develop?

_____

_____

#86 Break it Down

When you have a development goal, start by breaking it into smaller chunks.

For example, "I want to develop my communication skills" is too big a goal. Instead, think about what is it about your communications skills you want to develop and why. Is there a particular audience you want to communicate with more effectively?

Where do you feel you would most benefit from development?

- - - - - - - - - - - - - - - - - - - -

Describe what it would look and feel like if you were great at this area:

- - - - - - - - - - - - - - - - - - - -

What would be the outcomes of you being great at this?

- - - - - - - - - - - - - - - - - - - -

Why would it help your work wellness to develop it?

- - - - - - - - - - - - - - - - - - - -

Pick one small aspect of the area you chose. What could you work on to improve your overall level in this area?

- - - - - - - - - - - - - - - - - - - -

What action can you take to work on this?

- - - - - - - - - - - - - - - - - - - -

#87 Keep a Development Journal

Once you've put together one to three areas of developmental focus, keep track of your progress by writing in a development journal.

Create your template here (some questions are provided as an example, but feel free to add to or change these):

Developmental focus:

- What I did this week to advance this:

- What was the impact?

- How do I feel about this area?

- What will I focus on next week?

What other questions will you ask yourself weekly?

1. ⎯⎯⎯ ⎯ ⎯⎯ ⎯⎯⎯⎯ ⎯ ⎯⎯ ⎯⎯ ⎯ ⎯⎯

2. ⎯⎯⎯⎯⎯⎯⎯⎯ ⎯⎯⎯⎯⎯⎯ ⎯⎯ ⎯⎯⎯⎯

3. ⎯⎯ ⎯ ⎯⎯ ⎯ ⎯⎯ ⎯⎯ ⎯ ⎯⎯⎯

4. ⎯⎯⎯⎯⎯⎯⎯⎯ ⎯⎯⎯⎯⎯

5. ⎯⎯ ⎯ ⎯⎯ ⎯⎯⎯ ⎯ ⎯⎯ ⎯⎯ ⎯ ⎯⎯

6. ⎯⎯⎯⎯⎯⎯⎯ ⎯⎯⎯⎯⎯

7. ⎯⎯⎯ ⎯ ⎯⎯ ⎯⎯⎯ ⎯ ⎯ ⎯⎯ ⎯

#88 Find a Peer Mentor or Coach

It's unlikely you're the only one at your level who wants to develop. One connective way to blossom at work is to find a buddy who's also interested in their personal and professional growth (if you're self-employed, you may know others in your network in a similar position), and share what you're working on. Take turns to encourage, question and explore what they want to develop and let them do the same for you. Swap experience and ideas.

Who might be my learning buddy? Why this person?

What can I offer as a learning buddy?

What qualities can I bring to this kind of relationship?

#89 Share Knowledge

You'd be surprised at what you know that others don't. Connecting with others and sharing your experience can be a great way for you to grow. You can create an informal knowledge-sharing group which meets over lunch, or offer to share about a topic in which you have expertise on in your team meeting.

What topics are you an expert on that others aren't? Write a topic in each of the stars on this page.

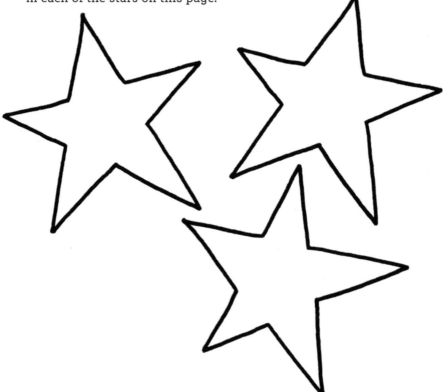

If you're stuck, ask a friend – you might be surprised at what they think you're an expert on!

#90 Grow Your Ability to Handle Emotions

Your personal growth is as important to your work wellness as your professional growth. Emotional intelligence – your ability to identify, understand and manage your and others' emotions in positive ways – is a sometimes neglected area of development that can give you a boost in your personal lives as well as at work.

When was the last time you felt emotional at work? (i.e. anger, frustration, sadness, annoyance, excitement, anxiety, pride, happiness, satisfaction, etc.)

- -

What was the emotion?

- -

What happened?

- -

How did you behave?

- -

What did you feel?

- -

Why did the situation create those feelings?

- -

What could you do differently next time to use or manage your emotions more effectively?

- -

(Examples might include using breathing techniques, journaling, taking a time out for five minutes and adapting your body language.)

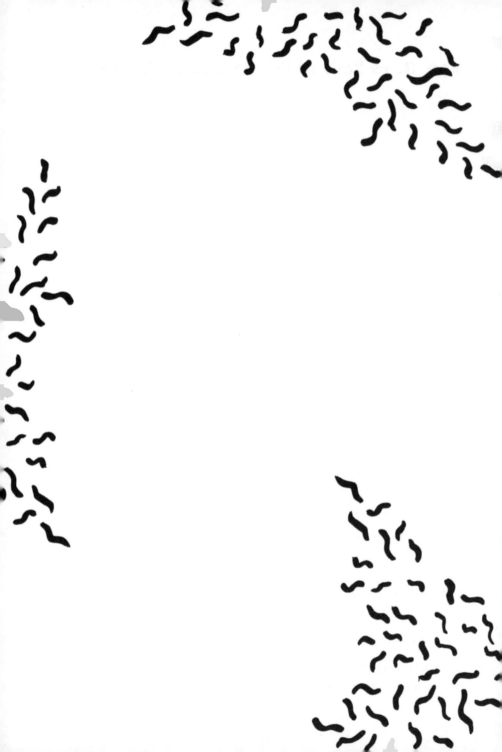

CHAPTER 10

Handling Change

Handling Change

We only have to look at the past few years to see how incredibly and quickly the world can change around us and, as individuals, there is little we can do about much of it (see **#20 Serenity Prayer**).

In work, the ability to adapt to change and be resilient is a hugely sought after quality in employees, and it will help us at a personal level as well as a professional level, given the huge number of changes we may face at work. Retirement, redundancy, coming back from extended leave (e.g. maternity leave or illness), moving jobs within the organization, moving to another organization or changing our boss are all types of change we may face.

Change can be difficult because it is often outside our control, and it's ambiguous, in that we don't always know what will happen after the change. In addition, we tend to focus on the negative aspects of potential change (as per our hardwiring – see **#11 One Positive Interaction a Day**) and it often feels safer to stick with what we know.

Whatever the change, hiding isn't going to work in the world we live in, whereas engaging with it and taking action is likely to help us face it more effectively and flourish while we do so.

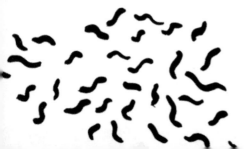

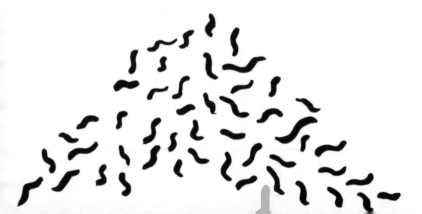

What you will find in this chapter

In this chapter, we look at the best ways to do exactly that. We **#91 Do a SWOT Analysis on the Change**, considering the strengths, weaknesses, opportunities and threats you may face as part of any modifications in circumstances. Once you have that analysis, you can ask yourself **#92 What Do You Need to Learn?**

Next it's time to **#93 Address the Stress**, in part by taking the time to **#94 Share Your Fears** and also by taking the opportunity to **#95 Make a Plan**.

We make room for what's coming when we **#96 Create a Release Ritual**, and then we get practical and face our fears in **#97 The Worst That Can Happen**. Next up, we **#98 Practise Reframing** and consider ideas on how to **#99 Handle Non-Work Issues and Change**.

Lastly, we remind ourselves of the simplest technique to give ourselves a moment of respite whatever we're facing: **#100 One Deep Breath**.

#91 Do a SWOT Analysis on the Change

When facing a change to your circumstances, it can help to analyse it and understand it better. You can use the "SWOT" tool to do this. SWOT stands for Strengths, Weaknesses, Opportunities and Threats.

Consider the change you are facing. Describe it here:

- -

- -

What are all the strengths, weaknesses, opportunities and threats that you face due to the change?

• What are your potential **Strengths** in this situation?	• What are your potential **Weaknesses** in this situation?
• What **Opportunities** might this situation bring you?	• What **Threats** might this situation pose to you?

#92 What Do You Need to Learn?

Once you've understood the scope of the change, how it might affect you and in what ways, think about where you might need to invest time in your development to rise up and successfully meet the challenges it brings.

List three areas relevant to the change where you could develop your skills:

1. _____

2. _____

3. _____

How could you build these skills?

_____

How does it feel to identify these potential growth areas?

_____

How confident are you that you could grow in these aspects?

_____

If necessary, what/whose help could you enlist?

_____

#93 Address the Stress

Change opens up the unknown and this brings up anxieties for most of us. Even though it can feel scary, identifying these fears can help us to create action to address them.

It's also helpful to use the ideas in the **#20 Serenity Prayer** to identify which fears you can address and which are out of your control right now.

Consider the fears that come up when you think about the change. Sort them into fears you can address (inner circle) and fears that are outside of your control (outer circle).

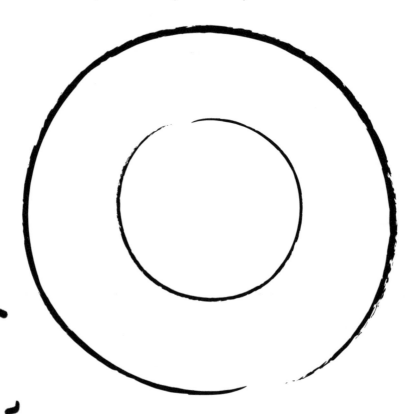

#94 Share Your Fears

You're not the first person to experience change, or even the specific change you're going through – others are likely to have faced it before.

Seek out a person, community, online group, book, podcast or any resource that helps to show you you're not alone in facing this kind of change. Write down what you have learned from reviewing this resource here:

How have others coped with this change?

What kinds of behaviours have others tried that didn't work and what can you learn from this?

What one action could you do this week to support you through this change?

#95 Make a Plan

Once you've understood the change and how it might impact you, and you've explored some possible ways to deal with it, it's time to make a plan that will enable you not only to face this change, but also to thrive as a result.

Focusing purely on the aspects that are within your ability to affect, create a plan of next steps. Start with the end in mind (e.g. if you are on maternity leave and the change is going back to work, then start from where you are now, with being back at work as your end goal).

What do I want to happen as a result of this change?

_____ _____

_____ _____

_____ _____

Where am I now in relation to this change?

— — — — — — — — — — —

— — — — — — — — — —

What are the timelines for this change?

· - · - · - · - · - · - · - · - · - · - · - · - -

- · - · - · - — - · - · - · - · - · - · - · - ·

- · - · - · - · - · - · - · - · - · - · - · - ·

What can I take action on?

_____

_____

What milestones can I break my progress toward my end goal into?

_____   _____

_____   _____

What actions and tasks will I need to do for each milestone?

_____   _____

_____   _____

What resources will I need?

_____   _____

_____   _____

How will I know when I am successful?

_____

_____

How do I feel about this change now I have a plan?

_____

#96 Create a Release Ritual

Sometimes, in order to let new opportunities into our life, we have to let go of some hopes and dreams before the change comes along.

To do this, it can be helpful to create a ritual to release those outdated ideas, so you have room for what's coming. It doesn't have to be complex, but you need to imbue it with meaning and structure.

Create a ritual to release the aspects of yourself that are no longer relevant. This will help you transition into the change.

1. Pick a place, a time and whatever props (such as a candle or scent) help you to feel grounded. You might want to choose coloured pens and pretty paper to write your old hopes and dreams on.

2. Let part of the ritual include writing down a description or drawing a representation of the "you" that existed before the change.

3. Then, as part of your ritual, thank this old self, then let this go in some way – whether by tearing it up, throwing it away or burning it.

4. Jot down your notes to prepare yourself for your own unique ritual opposite, so you can use it again in the future when you face change.

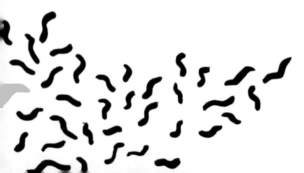

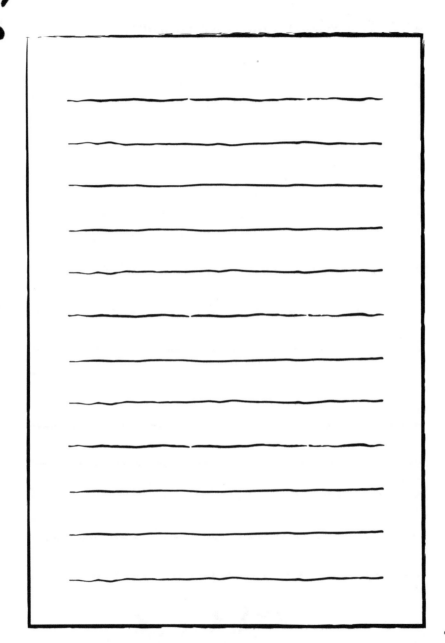

#97 The Worst That Can Happen

In relation to the change you are facing, thinking about the worst that can happen seems counter-intuitive, but facing your fears and being pragmatic about the future can actually help to relieve any anxiety you may have about it.

Fears tend to be more frightening when they are vague or unexplored rather than specific, and so not only will exploring them in this way give you some perspective on how realistic your fears are, but it will also help you to know what you're facing, so you can make a plan as to how you will deal with the worst scenario in the (unlikely) event it happens.

What are the worst possible negative consequences of this change?

How would you deal with it if the worst happened?

How realistic are the scenarios you've outlined here?

#98 Practise Reframing

In **#92 What Do You Need to Learn?** you identified the opportunities that might be present for you as part of the change. You've also identified your fears and the worst that can happen. Now it's time to consider some other possible interpretations of the situation to broaden your perspective and consider other ways to look at it.

What's your current interpretation of how this change will affect you?

Write down three different interpretations of the same situation:

1.

2.

3.

#99 Handle Non-Work Issues

Our personal lives and work lives aren't as distinct as we would like them to be. Change outside of work – a divorce, a break-up, moving house, looking after an elderly parent, sick children – all these can cause worries that affect our work.

Depending on the severity of the issue, you can approach them in different ways, for example:

- Talk to your boss (even if you're the boss!) and take a short time off – part of your holiday, or if you're with a business, they might have other ways of handling it such as bereavement leave

- Take "worry breaks" during the day. Give your worry your full attention during those times and park it for the remainder

Experiment with "worry breaks".

Pick an issue you have some mild anxiety or worry about.

Schedule in two ten-minute breaks today when you will "worry" about it. Apart from this time, put it to the back of your mind. If you find yourself thinking about it, tell yourself firmly that "I'm going to worry about that at 3pm" or whenever you have next decided to worry.

After your worry break, journal here on how it went:

— — — — — — — — — — — —

— — — — — — — — — — — —

— — — — — — — — — — — —

#100 One Deep Breath

Finally, don't discount the power of your breath. You don't have to meditate for hours to gain the benefits of connecting with your breath. Taking a moment to do this exercise will help you stop for a moment and short-circuit some of the anxiety you might be feeling, as well as ground you in your body, rather than being consumed by racing thoughts. This exercise is useful when change overwhelms us, or when any situation gets difficult or challenging. Or, indeed, it can be a simple work wellness practice to include throughout your day.

1. Put both feet on the ground.

2. Put your hand over your heart and close your eyes.

3. Breathe in slowly and deeply for a count of four.

4. Breathe out slowly and from your abdomen for a count of eight. Imagine your breath being pushed out and down toward the floor, through your feet.

5. Repeat for as long as you like.

Final Thoughts

In closing

The ideas in this book are designed to support you in being your best self at work.

Try them out, but remember to be gentle with yourself as you do. Don't try everything at once and treat them as experiments to enjoy.

Remember that to *be* your best self at work, you have to *bring* your best self to work, which means taking care of yourself *outside* work as much as you do *in* work.

You might also be interested in picking up my other book, *This Is For You: A Creative Toolkit for Better Self-Care*, to support you in this.

Be kind to yourself,
Ellen x

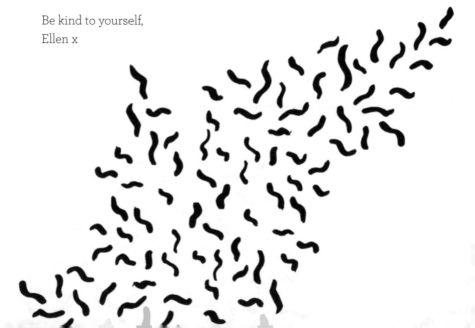

Acknowledgements

I am so grateful to all the wonderful work psychologists, HR professionals and coaches I have known and learned from over my 20-plus years of work. The community is a kind and supportive one, and I've been lucky to have worked with so many knowledgeable people.

I also want to thank my editor. Anya Hayes at Watkins has been warm and receptive to my ideas. I appreciate her calmness and positivity, despite my challenges along the way. I love the way Watkins Publishing brings my work to life.

My family are hugely supportive, especially my godmothers Ellen Dunne and Anne Bard, who are always ready to provide a listening ear. My sister, Sarah Bard, is a wonderful cheerleader, and my mother, Mary Bard, is always happy to give her pragmatic view on ideas to help them work better for the reader and she provided invaluable support as I wrote the book.

Friends Dr Anna Charbonneau and Graham Morley reminded me to keep an eye on my own self-care while writing.

Lastly, I am incredibly grateful to my Fox and small-Fox, who ground me in a way I never thought I'd experience through being part of a little family. For helping me to live our values, for support with the book, for being a truly amazing life partner, I thank you. This book would not exist without you.

Further Reading

The following titles are loosely sorted into categories, though most books are relevant to several areas.

1. Physical Environment
Joy at Work, Marie Kondo
*Unf**k Your Habitat*, Rachel Hoffman

2. Mindset
7 Habits of Highly Effective People, Stephen Covey
Mindset, Carol Dweck

3. Working in a Home Office
Outer Order, Inner Calm, Gretchen Rubin
The Joy of Being Selfish: Why You Need Boundaries and How to Set Them, Michelle Elman

4. Doing the Hard Stuff
The Mind Map Book, Tony Buzan
Atomic Habits, James Clear

5. Productivity and Focus
Getting Things Done, David Allen
Deep Work, Cal Newport

6. Work Breaks
Play, Stuart Brown
Why We Sleep, Matthew Walker

7. Time Management
When, Daniel Pink
12-Week Year, Brian P. Moran

8. Work Relationships
Emotional Agility, Susan David
Give and Take, Adam Grant

9. Progression and Development
Emotional Intelligence, Daniel Goleman
Daring Greatly, Brene Brown

10. Handling Change
Resilient, Rick Hanson
59 seconds, Richard Wiseman

This edition published in the UK and USA 2022 by
Watkins, an imprint of Watkins Media Limited
Unit 11, Shepperton House, 83–93 Shepperton Road
London N1 3DF

enquiries@watkinspublishing.com

Commissioning Editor: Anya Hayes
Editor: Victoria Godden
Editorial Assistant: Brittany Willis
Art Director: Georgina Hewitt
Designer: Steven Williamson
Production: Uzma Taj

Printed in United Kingdom by TJ Books

A CIP record for this book is available from the British Library

ISBN: 978-1-78678-596-1

10 9 8 7 6 5 4 3 2 1

www.watkinspublishing.com

NB: I am not a medical doctor, and the content of this book is not intended to be
a substitute for medical advice, diagnosis or treatment. Always seek the advice
of your physician or other appropriately qualified health provider with questions
regarding a medical condition. Seeing a doctor, or a therapist, is an act that will
support your work wellness!

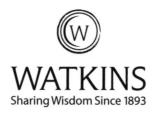

WATKINS

Sharing Wisdom Since 1893

The story of Watkins began in 1893, when scholar of esotericism John Watkins founded our bookshop, inspired by the lament of his friend and teacher Madame Blavatsky that there was nowhere in London to buy books on mysticism, occultism or metaphysics. That moment marked the birth of Watkins, soon to become the publisher of many of the leading lights of spiritual literature, including Carl Jung, Rudolf Steiner, Alice Bailey and Chögyam Trungpa.

Today, the passion at Watkins Publishing for vigorous questioning is still resolute. Our stimulating and groundbreaking list ranges from ancient traditions and complementary medicine to the latest ideas about personal development, holistic wellbeing and consciousness exploration. We remain at the cutting edge, committed to publishing books that change lives.

DISCOVER MORE AT:

www.watkinspublishing.com

Read our blog

Watch and listen to
our authors in action

Sign up to
our mailing list

We celebrate conscious, passionate, wise and happy living.

Be part of that community by visiting

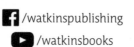 /watkinspublishing

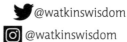 @watkinswisdom

/watkinsbooks

@watkinswisdom